10·11·79

Stay young
at heart

Stay young
at heart

John Davis Cantwell, MD

Nelson-Hall
 Chicago

Library of Congress Cataloging in Publication Data

Cantwell, John D
    Stay young at heart.

      Bibliography: p.
      Includes index.
      1.   Heart—Diseases—Prevention.   2.   Exercise—
Physiological effect.   I.   Title.
RC682.C36   616.1'2'05   75-25958
ISBN 0-88229-247-1

Copyright © 1975 by John Davis Cantwell

Manufactured in the United States of America.

To

The men and women in the
cardiac rehabilitation program
at Georgia Baptist Hospital,
whose faith, courage, and determination
are a constant stimulus to me.

Contents

Preface

Stay young at heart! The words have been used in other connotations, but the emphasis in this book is clearly on health and diseases of the heart.

It is concerned with one particular disease, with the factors which seem to influence the disease, and with ways in which the malady can be approached from a preventive standpoint, based on sound scientific principles.

Coronary atherosclerotic heart disease, better known as coronary thrombosis, heart attack, or hardening of the arteries, is a problem of enormous magnitude in the United States and in some other parts of the world. It is largely because of this disease that American men rank thirty-fifth on the list of life expectancy (United Nations Statistics).

Life expectancy for men

Top 6	Years	Bottom 6	Years
1. Sweden	71.9	Central African Republic	33.0
2. Norway	71.0	Upper Volta	32.1
3. Iceland	70.8	Togo	31.6
4. Netherlands	70.7	Chad	29.0
5. Denmark	70.7	Guinea	26.0
6. Israel	70.7	Gabon	25.0
35. USA	66.6		

Heart disease is increasingly becoming a problem for women, who were once thought to have some obscure protection prior to the time of menopause. A Brooklyn pathologist reported that during the decade of 1949–1959 there were twelve sudden coronary deaths for men for every one death in women. During the four-year period from 1967 through 1971, this ratio had dwindled to 4:1, and was closely correlated with increased cigarette smoking by women.

Although the specific cause of coronary heart disease is not known, many factors besides cigarette smoking are associated with an increased risk of premature coronary disease, that is, disease prior to age fifty-five. Coronary risk factors were lucidly described in Dr. Jeremiah Stamler's book, *Your Heart Has Nine Lives*. One significant risk factor mentioned in his book is Americans' lack of physical activity. As a nation we are lazy and soft. Approximately forty-five percent or 49 million of 109 million American men and women do not engage in physical activity for exercise, according to a research survey prompted by the President's Council on Physical Fitness. Of the 60 million Americans who did exercise, two-thirds did nothing more strenuous than walking; yet these people felt that they were getting sufficient exercise! Sadly, some 80 percent of the adults surveyed stated that they had never been advised by a physician to exercise regularly.

Since the publication of Dr. Stamler's book and the popular book about exercise by Dr. Kenneth Cooper, *Aerobics,* a great deal has been said about exercise and heart disease. The purpose of this book is to publicize what is currently known about heart disease and American lifestyles. It begins with an overview of scientific data pertaining to coronary disease and to the various risk factors, emphasizing the effects of sedentary living on the cardiovascular system. The nuances of exercise stress testing and a new method of prescribing exercise for the general public are presented. Individual coronary risk factors other than inadequate exercise—hypertension, high blood cholesterol, and cigarette smoking—are covered in detail. Finally, preventive cardiology practices in childhood will be highlighted along with results of a preventive cardiology clinic.

It is the author's hope that this book will stimulate the seemingly healthy person to take a closer look at himself (or herself) and to modify his or her lifestyle for maximum health.

Acknowledgments

I would like to express my appreciation to Edward W. Watt, who has been a source of inspiration to me in our clinical practice. Dr. Watt's article on obesity was a useful reference for Chapter 15, and he compiled the statistical data for Chapter 19. I would also like to thank Dr. Gerald Fletcher for encouraging me in the pursuit of preventive cardiology and Dr. Fred L. Allman, Jr., for his help and support in organizing the Preventive Cardiology Clinic.

Bob Beveridge did the photography, and Neaka Kooken was the typist. I appreciate their efforts.

I would like to pay tribute to my father, Dr. Arthur A. Cantwell, and my uncle, Dr. Roger C. Cantwell, whose love for medicine was exceeded only by their love for their patients and for life itself.

Coronary heart disease in perspective

The World Health Organization recently issued the following statement:

Coronary heart disease has reached enormous proportions, striking more and more at younger subjects. It will result in coming years in the greatest epidemic mankind has faced unless we are able to reverse the trend by concentrated research into its cause and prevention.

Most people today are aware of the problem. Coronary heart disease causes nearly 40 percent of all deaths in the United States. When one includes related vascular disease, strokes, and hypertension, the figure increases to over 50 percent.

Autopsy studies of young men and women who died in automobile and plane accidents and in the Korean and Vietnam wars have consistently shown that atherosclerosis—thickening and hardening of the arterial walls—begins very early in life. Three percent of nearly 300 American soldiers killed in Korea had almost total occlusion—blocking—of one major coronary artery. Twenty percent had more than half of one major artery blocked. Of 105 United States soldiers killed in Vietnam, with a mean age of twenty-two, 45 percent had some evidence of atherosclerosis, and five percent had severe coronary atherosclerosis.

Forty-one servicemen, all under forty, volunteered for coronary arteriograms because of a family history of coronary heart disease or high blood fat levels, although they themselves had shown no signs or symptoms of cardiac disease. This study, the first of its kind, was conducted by Dr. Carl J. Pepine, Director of the Cardiac Catheterization Laboratory of the Philadelphia Naval Hospital. Nineteen of the men had at least half of a coronary vessel occluded, while one-fourth of the men had at least two diseased coronary arteries. Most of these men were quite active physically, running several miles per day. Paradoxically, the man with the most extensive disease ran five miles per day and had successfully completed three tours of duty in Vietnam. In a follow-up two and one-half years later, three of the nineteen men had suffered heart attacks.

Marvelous advances in the diagnosis and treatment of coronary disease have been made during the past decade. Diagnostic advances include the ability to screen individuals for different combinations of fats in the blood—abnormal amounts of cholesterol and triglyceride. For instance, one blood fat pattern (Type IV—high triglyceride, normal cholesterol) is better treated with a low carbohydrate diet than one low in fats. Other advances have been made in exercise stress testing, where computerized methods have added refinement to the identification of an abnormal electrocardiogram.

The most dramatic development, however, has been the technique of coronary arteriography. A catheter is inserted in an arm or leg blood vessel and positioned into one of the coronary arteries. Dye is thus injected and films are made, enabling us to determine the distribution and degree of coronary atherosclerosis (Figure 1–1). Using other techniques

Figure 1–1 Diagram of cardiac catheterization.

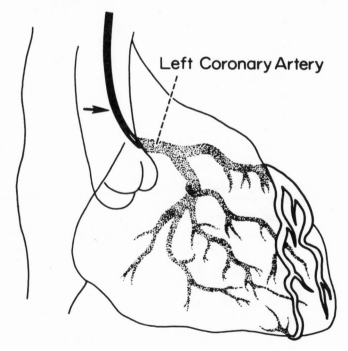

Left Coronary Artery

of cardiac catheterization, we can also determine how well the heart muscle itself is functioning. The functioning of the heart can be illustrated by the analogy of water flow through pipes to a faucet. It is detrimental to the overall system if the diameter of the pipes is narrowed by 75 percent. It is more so if, in addition to the narrowing of the pipes (coronary artery), the faucet (heart muscle) is malfunctioning.

In the treatment of coronary disease, there have been major advances in both medical and surgical approaches. New drugs are available to treat high blood pressure and high blood fats (cholesterol and triglycerides). New drugs are also available to treat chest pain related to coronary insufficiency (angina pectoris), including Isordil, a coronary vasodilator, and Inderal, a drug which reduces the oxygen requirement of heart muscle. The hospital structure has been altered, giving us specific coronary and intensive care units wherein specialized equipment and personnel are immediately available and where surveillance is continuous. Medically supervised programs of exercise, prescribed for and carried out by coronary patients, represent a significant advance.

The drama of surgery has a way of capturing headlines, and such has been the case in the field of cardiovascular surgery. The most exciting development has been the use of the saphenous vein grafts to construct detours around narrow or occluded coronary arteries. The proximal portion of the vein graft (obtained from the inner thigh region) is sewn into the base of the aorta, while the distal portion is connected to the area of the coronary artery beyond the obstruction (Figure 1–2). Heart transplants had a

Figure 1–2 Detour around narrow artery.

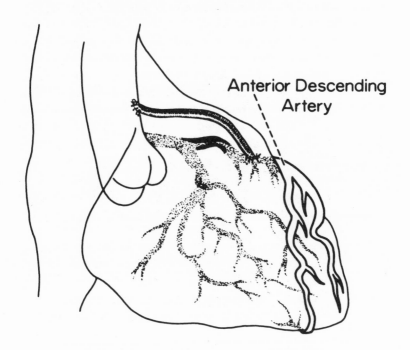

Anterior Descending Artery

brief surge of popularity, but proved disappointing and need further study and assessment.

Despite the medical and surgical advances and despite coronary care units and specialized ambulance teams, several facts continue to cause concern:

1. 60 percent of the deaths from coronary heart disease occur suddenly, before the patient can get to the physician or the hospital.
2. The death rate—16–33 percent—while in the hospital remains high.

3. Of persons who survive an initial myocardial infarction, recurrence rates have remained appreciable.
4. The long-term effects of new surgical procedures are completely unknown. For instance, will a significant proportion of the vein grafts themselves develop degenerative disease over a five to ten year period?

While the diagnosis and treatment of disease is obviously important, the prevention of disease clearly makes the most sense. It is possible to prevent or to markedly decrease the prevalence of a disease long before the specific cause (or causes) of that disease are known.

2

Coronary risk factors

Considerable research has been devoted to identifying factors that are characteristic of individuals who develop coronary heart disease. Studies were set up as long as twenty years ago in Framingham, Massachusetts, Tecumseh, Michigan, and Chicago, Illinois, to evaluate large groups of people. Records were kept of persons who developed coronary disease, and compared to those of another group who did not. Ten coronary risk factors were identified from these prolonged studies. The first three listed are probably the most important, as will be explained later in this chapter.

1. Blood fat abnormalities (increased cholesterol and/or triglyceride levels)
2. High blood pressure
3. Cigarette smoking

4. Diabetes mellitus
5. Physical inactivity
6. Overweight (and overfat)
7. Diet (level of saturated fat intake)
8. Heredity
9. Personality and behavior patterns
10. Disorders in blood coagulation

Of course, age is another important factor, and sex too, particularly among Caucasians.

Risk factors accumulate

The risk factors are cumulative; the more factors, the greater the chance of heart disease. According to Dr. Jeremiah Stamler of Northwestern University, if you have only one, chances of having a heart attack before age fifty-five range from one in twenty to one in fifty. If you have two risk factors, chances increase significantly—one in ten. If you have three or more, your chances are one in two!

This is probably an oversimplification, because certain risk factors carry more weight than others. In addition, the degree of each factor needs to be taken into account. A man who smokes cigarettes, has a serum cholesterol level greater than 250 mg and high blood pressure, has an eight and one-half times greater chance of developing a coronary attack than the man with none of these (Figure 2–1).

Which factors are most important?

It has been difficult to ascertain the relative importance of the various risk factors among differ-

Figure 2–1

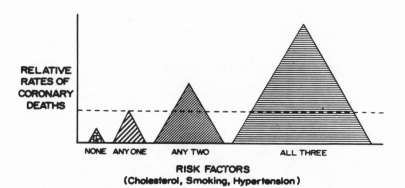

ent individuals and different cultural groups. For example, exercise would appear to be of great value among the tall and strong Masai warriors of East Africa, who have hardly any atherosclerosis despite a diet high in saturated fat. Exercise levels might also explain the difference between Irishmen in Ireland and their brothers who migrated to the Boston area. In Ireland, the men consumed more calories and saturated fat than they did in the United States. Yet they had a significantly lower incidence of coronary disease. The difference again might be exercise. Still other studies have shown that regular exercise is certainly no guarantee against premature coronary disease. The Rendille tribe of northern Kenya, who walk for miles each day, still have a high incidence of atherosclerosis. This might be due to their diet, which is high in saturated animal fat. But so is the diet of the Masai. If diet is more important than physical activity, however, how can one explain the Masai?

Although certain risk factors are probably more

ominous than others, *all* of the risk factors need to be considered for any one person. One cannot balance one factor against another. For example, exercise does not negate the deleterious effects of cigarette smoking. During military duty in the United States Public Health Service, I treated eight American prisoners who suffered heart attacks while still in their thirties. In looking at their risk factors, I noticed that the average number of positive factors per man was 5.2. Three of the prisoners had exercised vigorously on a daily basis for up to three years prior to having an attack. This offered little protection in the face of cigarette smoking, personality and behavior pattern abnormalities, dietary indiscretion, and the like.

One solution to the problem of trying to compare data from different studies was to use the same procedures in gathering information and having the analysis and interpretation performed by a single group of physicians. One such study was performed under the direction of Dr. Ancel Keys, a research specialist at the University of Minnesota, in seven countries—Japan, Greece, Yugoslavia, Italy, the Netherlands, Finland, and the United States. A sample population of more than 12,000 men was studied. The various risk factors were analyzed, using special mathematical equations, and all other measured factors were held constant while a single factor was being assessed.

Results

Japan had the lowest rate of coronary heart disease, while the United States and Finland had the highest. Levels of physical activity could perhaps explain the low rates in the Japanese, who tend to be very active, and the high rates for affluent Americans, but certainly not the high rates among the Finns, who represent the ultimate in physical fitness orientation.

In this study, the following three risk factors seemed to correlate best with high rates of coronary heart disease:

> High blood cholesterol
> High blood pressure
> Diet high in saturated animal fats

Cigarette smoking must also be considered a major coronary risk factor in view of almost overwhelming evidence from other studies, even though close correlations were not seen in the Seven Countries Study. Body weight and body fat levels were less significant. Unfortunately, personality and behavior patterns were not tested, nor were blood coagulation studies reported. Moreover, leisure time physical activity was not ascertained, and hence it would be unfair to consider it as a less significant risk factor in this study.

Can anything be done? Given the identification and importance of the various risk factors, is there any evidence that a change or reduction of risk factors will lower the chances of coronary heart disease or prevent recurrences of coronary attacks?

Prevention studies

Results of multiple studies are now available that offer some answers to the problem of preventing the primary coronary event (either sudden death, angina pectoris [chest pain due to coronary disease], or a myocardial infarction [heart attack]).

The New York anti-coronary club

Nine hundred and forty-one men, aged forty to fifty-nine with no evidence of coronary disease, began a dietary study in 1957. A control group of 457 men of similar age was assembled in 1959. The two groups were rather well-matched with respect to blood cholesterol levels and cigarette smoking. The experimental group, who tended to have higher levels of body fat and blood pressure, were placed on a low-calorie, low-fat diet. The control group simply continued eating what they had been accustomed to. During the ten-year follow-up period, those on the special diet achieved moderate weight reduction and an average reduction of serum cholesterol of 30 mg percent—a moderately good reduction. Despite the fact that they were a higher risk to begin with (more obesity and hypertension than the control group), the rate of coronary disease development was less than half that of the control group.

The Los Angeles Veterans Administration study

In another dietary study 590 men with a median age of sixty-five, all free of heart disease, were assigned to two groups at random. The groups were comparable in terms of risk factors such as blood cholesterol level and blood pressure. Two separate food lines were set up in the VA facility.

One food line provided a diet low in saturated fats and cholesterol and high in polyunsaturated fat intake. In the other cafeteria line there was no attempt to reduce the total level of saturated and polyunsaturated fat. Neither line restricted or reduced the usual daily caloric intake of the men. The study was "double blind" in the sense that the patients were not told which line constituted the study diet, nor were the physicians analyzing the data aware of which line of food an individual used. Those on the special diet experienced an average decrease of 12.7 percent in blood cholesterol levels. More significantly, after eight years of study, those on the special diet had only one-third the incidence of myocardial infarction, sudden death due to coronary disease, and cerebrovascular events compared to the control group.

The Finnish mental hospital study

Patients from two mental hospitals in Helsinki participated in still another diet study to see whether a change in saturated fat intake would reduce the risk of coronary disease. Patients from Hospital N, 234 men with a mean age of 51.4 years, were placed on a low saturated fat diet in 1959. One hundred and seventy-two men from Hospital K, matched with Hospital N patients in age, hypertension, and cigarette smoking, served as the control group. Over a six-year period, the serum cholesterol level fell an average of 21.2 mg percent in the patients on the special diet. The annual incidence of coronary heart disease, as determined electrocardiographically, was over two times higher in the control group. At the end of six years, the hospital patients switched diets.

Hence, Hospital N was now on the control diet while Hospital K was on the special diet. With reversal of diets, a similar reversal of serum cholesterol levels was noted. The effect of the diet switch on the incidence of coronary heart disease, however, has not been tabulated as yet.

The Chicago coronary preventive evaluation program

The Chicago study, involving 519 men with ages ranging from forty to fifty-nine, began in 1958. As in the three previous studies, these men were judged to be free from coronary disease at the beginning of the study. Unlike the three previous studies, which dealt only with dietary intervention, the Chicago program focused on the correction of five coronary risk factors—high blood cholesterol, high blood pressure, obesity, physical inactivity, and cigarette smoking. The individuals were studied over a seven-year period and were compared with a control group of 2916 men who were roughly comparable in terms of age and risk factors. The control group had seven times the incidence of sudden death, four times the incidence of death caused by coronary disease, and twice the total mortality rate of the study group. Of those who dropped out of the special study group, rates of sudden death and deaths from coronary disease were five times higher than in those who adhered to the risk-factor reduction program.

The Veterans Administration study on antihypertensive drugs

Three hundred eighty patients with mild to moderate high blood pressure (diastolic pressure ranging

from 90 mm Hg to 114 mm Hg) were randomly assigned to two groups. The groups were comparable in
age, duration of hypertension, serum cholesterol
level, race, ECG, and chest X-ray findings. Using a
double blind technique, one group received an active
drug program to lower blood pressure while the
other was treated with placebos. Over a five-year
period, the incidence of coronary artery disease was
slightly less in the treated group than in the placebo
group. The difference had no statistical significance.
However, in the group treated there were no instances of congestive heart failure (impaired ability
of the heart to maintain adequate blood flow to the
tissues), as compared to eleven cases in the control
group. Moreover, the incidence of strokes was four
times greater in the control group than in the treated
group.

Although additional studies are in progress, the
five studies here have all illustrated the same general
trend—namely, that an aggressive attack on major
coronary risk factors (diet, hypertension, and serum
cholesterol), can result in significant decreases in
cardiovascular events.

Studies of recurrence rates

What about the individual who has already suffered a heart attack or chest pain (angina
pectoris) due to coronary insufficiency? Is it possible
to use the same therapy to decrease the chances of
a second heart attack and to prolong life?

The Oslo diet-heart study

A group of 412 men, aged thirty to sixty-four,

comprised this study. These men had been discharged from various hospitals in the Norwegian city between 1956–1958, all with a diagnosis of a myocardial infarction. By a random process, the men were divided into two groups comparable in terms of age, serum cholesterol, and severity of coronary disease. Members of Group A were placed on a diet low in cholesterol and animal fats and rich in vegetable oil. The control Group B made no modifications in their routine diet, which was relatively high in those foods which contain saturated animal fat (eggs, whole milk, butter, beef, and cheese).

After the first five years of the study, the mean reduction of serum cholesterol was 17.6 percent in the diet group and 3.7 percent in the control group. After eleven years those in the diet group experienced a lower death rate from myocardial infarction than did the control.

When data from both groups were combined, a significant observation was made. For individuals who smoked cigarettes, had high blood cholesterol, and high blood pressure, the death rate from recurrent myocardial infarction was three times greater than for those individuals lacking these characteristics. It should be emphasized that these three risk factors can be controlled by abstention, diet, and drugs. It should also be noted that this study did not include attempts to decrease more than the dietary factor. Additional studies of the combined approach against multiple risk factors, such as the primary prevention study in Chicago, are forthcoming.

The Montclair study

Another secondary prevention study involving

dietary management was carried out by the Atherosclerotic Research Group, St. Vincent's Hospital,
Montclair, New Jersey. Two hundred men, aged
thirty to fifty, with prior myocardial infarctions,
were divided into a diet and a control group. Again
the groups were similar in regard to age, number of
myocardial infarctions, blood pressure, and serum
cholesterol levels. Death rates from myocardial *re*infarction over a five-year period were significantly
lower for those on the low saturated fat diet who
were also under forty-five. The death rate reduction
among those over forty-five was less striking. This
would suggest that the earlier in life that dietary
changes are made, the more effective they are in
preventing myocardial infarction.

Conclusion

In summary, let us briefly review the
salient points of the studies previously described:

First—A number of factors have been identified
which cause an individual to become a higher risk
for coronary heart disease. At present, the factors of
greatest significance include *1)* diet high in saturated animal fats, *2)* high blood pressure, *3)* high
blood cholesterol and *4)* cigarette smoking.

Second—The risk factors are cumulative, meaning that the more factors one has, the greater is the
risk of a premature coronary event.

Third—It is currently possible to correct or at
least control each of the risk factors above.

Fourth—Studies involving normal persons consistently revealed that by altering at least one of the
risk factors, you can alter the rate of coronary disease development.

Fifth—Studies involving persons who have already experienced a myocardial infarction also indicate that by altering one of the risk factors, you can decrease the rate of recurrent myocardial infarction, particularly if you are under forty-five.

With this evidence and faced with an epidemic of coronary heart disease, it behooves us to utilize the available information now to decrease our own risk, and that of our children, of developing coronary atherosclerotic heart disease.

———

References to data can be found in *Exercise and Coronary Heart Disease*, Charles C. Thomas Co., Springfield, Ill., 1974 (J. D. Cantwell, M.D., and Gerald F. Fletcher, M.D., coauthors).

3

Sedentary living

In order to comprehend the effects of our sedentary lifestyle, we need to be familiar with epidemiology, the study of epidemic disease, its natural history, and those factors that may influence it. Many such studies have been carried out in an attempt to assess the impact of physical activity on coronary heart disease. In a lucid review of thirty-five reports of epidemiologic research relating to the alleged association between coronary heart disease and a sedentary lifestyle, Victor Froelicher categorized the research into four groups: *1)* retrospective studies, *2)* prospective studies, *3)* autopsy evaluations, and *4)* rehabilitation studies.

Retrospective studies

What is retrospective research? In brief, it is a study of persons who have already developed coronary heart disease which attempts to identify those factors in their past that might have predisposed them to the disease. Certainly one of the most famous studies of this type involved London bus employees, both drivers and conductors. In this study, Dr. Jerry Morris reviewed data on 31,000 men aged thirty-five to sixty-four. He discovered that the more sedentary bus drivers had one and a half times the rate of coronary disease as did the more active conductors. The moderately active conductors spent most of their day going up and down the steps of double-decked buses. Moreover, the sudden death rates and death rates during the first two months after a heart attack were twice as high in the drivers. This study has often formed the basis for the hard sell of the benefits of exercise by various enthusiasts. However, certain significant weaknesses in the study should be mentioned. For instance, there was no attempt to quantify levels of activity in the two groups, nor were studies made of their off-the-job activities. After the original results were published, it was learned that blood pressure, body weight, and blood cholesterol levels of the drivers were higher than those of the conductors. This difference apparently existed even at the time both groups first applied for their jobs. Such differences could have made the drivers higher risks for coronary disease for other reasons than physical activity levels.

A team of investigators at the University of Minnesota reported on death rates of American railroad workers in 1962. They discovered that the more active sectionmen, who laid track by hand as part of their job, had less than half the incidence of coronary disease as did the sedentary clerks. While it could be surmised from this that men in sedentary occupations have more coronary disease than those engaged in moderate to heavy physical activity, further analysis created problems. It seems that certain clerks actually used up more calories per day than the more active sectionmen. Additionally, some of the sectionmen transferred to clerical jobs subsequent to developing signs of coronary heart disease; this probably contributed to the higher coronary death rates. Thus, rather than postulating any protective effect of exercise, it is also possible to explain some of the differences by job transfers and retirement practices.

The ex-college athlete has been a favorite research subject for retrospective studies. Paul Dudley White, the internationally renowned heart specialist who was former President Eisenhower's doctor, was unable to detect any harmful cardiac effects of strenuous activity in a long-term study of former Harvard football players, conducted 25–50 years following their graduation. Indeed, he noted that those who remained physically active in later life had fewer heart attacks when compared to less active students. A study of 172 former (1882–1902) crew members at Harvard and Yale indicated a greater life span for the crew members (67.9 years) than for the non-athletic control group (61.6 years). However, in this study specific causes of death were difficult to ascertain; in many instances and when the cause of death prior to age sixty was known, there were no significant differences in heart attacks between the two groups.

Another study on athletes was performed by Peter Schnohr, a Danish cardiologist, who gathered information on 297 athletic champions born between 1880 and 1910. Dr. Schnohr compared their death rates with those of the general male population in

Denmark. He noticed that the causes of death were the same, but the former athletes had much less chance of dying before age fifty.

A recent publication dealing with longevity and cardiac death rates in 681 former Harvard lettermen showed that there were no significant differences in longevity when the athletes were subdivided by type of sport. However, George Sheehan, a New Jersey cardiologist, pointed out that it would have been more meaningful to subdivide the athletes by body build (somatype), for many feel that the ectomorph (tall, thin) has much less coronary risk than the mesomorph (short, muscular).

In a retrospective study of a somewhat different nature, 55,000 men aged twenty-five to sixty-four, who were enrolled in the Health Insurance Plan of New York, were evaluated. During a sixteen-month period, 301 men suffered heart attacks. Questionnaires and personal interviews were carried out with either the patient or his widow. Data on physical activity at work or during leisure hours were collected. This permitted classification of the men into activity groups of light, moderate, and heavy intensity. Of those in the light physical activity group, 49 percent died during the early phase of the heart disease as opposed to only 13 percent in the heavy activity group. Thus, it would appear that even if physical activity failed to prevent a heart attack, it could greatly increase one's chances of survival.

Prospective studies

In prospective studies, a population group is carefully evaluated and then followed closely over a period of time. Individuals who develop coro-

nary disease in the follow-up period are compared
with those who didn't, utilizing the medical information obtained from the initial and subsequent ex-
aminations wherever possible. A study of this kind
involved a sixteen-year follow-up on 3000 San Francisco longshoremen, aged thirty-five to sixty-four.
They were separated into two levels of work activity;
the two levels involved a difference of over 900
calories of energy expenditure per day. Over the
sixteen-year period, 291 men died of coronary disease. The death rate was 33 percent higher among
those in the less active group. It was evident that the
difference in activity level applied, even when levels
of blood pressure and cigarette-smoking were considered. A drawback to the study was that blood
cholesterol levels were not measured, causing specu-
lation as to whether or not this important risk factor
could have explained at least part of the differences.

The Seven Countries Study alluded to in Chapter
2 is a prospective study still in progress. When the
data were tabulated at the five-year point, there were
marked inconsistencies in physical activity levels and
coronary disease rates. For instance, Finland had the
highest rate of coronary disease and one of the highest rates of physical activity. However, rate of
physical activity was assumed rather than actually
measured (either by treadmill testing or work energy
expenditure determinations), and we must wait for
the final data before strong assumptions can be
made.

A study in Gothenburg, Sweden, has captured
the interest of cardiologists the world over. It involved 834 men all born in the year 1913. The men
were all thoroughly examined in 1963 when they
were fifty years old. None had clinical signs of coro-

nary heart disease at that time. They were divided into occupation activity classifications of heavy, medium, and light. Over the next four years, twenty-three of the men experienced heart attacks and eighteen men had the exertion-related chest pain known as angina pectoris. Interestingly, these episodes were significantly less frequent in the heavy activity group. Unfortunately, leisure time activities were not considered.

A recent report by cardiologist Jerry Morris did consider exercise habits during leisure hours. During the years 1968–1970, Dr. Morris and his team of investigators obtained weekend-activity questionnaires from over 16,000 middle-aged men—all of them executive-grade civil servants. Subsequent to the initial evaluations, 232 of the men have developed evidence of coronary disease. Those who reported vigorous activity during the two-day weekend assessed had only one-third the risk of developing coronary disease of those in the less active group. One significant shortcoming of this study is that the individuals' physical activity was sampled on a single weekend only. It is quite possible that a usually active sportsman was inactive that particular weekend due to an upper respiratory infection. Likewise, a sedentary person whose wife finally prodded him into completing a project in the basement that particular weekend would be falsely classified as being relatively active.

Pathological studies

An autopsy study conducted on athlete Clarence De Mar did much to deflate the theory that too much exercise is detrimental to the heart. De Mar was a remarkable man who competed in over 1000 long distance races during a sixty-year period, including over one hundred marathon races, thirty-four of which were in Boston. His record of seven victories in the marathon (cross-country footrace of twenty-six miles, 385 yards) has never been equalled. De Mar died of metastatic bowel cancer at age seventy, but on his death, pathologists found that the diameter of his coronary arteries was two to three times that of the average man in this age group. Although several areas of his coronary vessels showed hardening (atherosclerosis), the overall size of the arteries was such that this was of little consequence. It is not possible to exclude the chance that De Mar inherited larger than average coronary arteries; however, there is nothing in his family history to suggest this.

The second autopsy study of interest—the National British Autopsy Series of 1954–1956—included studies of 3800 men, aged forty-five to seventy, who had died of noncoronary causes. The occupations of the deceased were categorized as involving light, moderate, or heavy physical exertion. The degree of coronary artery narrowing was independently assessed. The pathologists reported that a "silent" occlusion of a major artery (that is, a complete occlusion without the patient's awareness) was more common in the light activity group.

Rehabilitation studies

The effect of exercise on coronary patients in preventing new cardiac problems has been reported from several major medical centers. From 1961 to 1966 Dr. Viktor Gottheiner conducted a five-year follow-up on over 1000 Israeli men with known coronary disease, all of whom participated in a variety of individual and team sports, including weight lifting and competitive games. He reported the death rate to be only 3.6 percent as compared to 12 percent for a comparable nonexercising group of Israelis with documented coronary disease.

In Cleveland, 100 postcoronary patients participated in a thrice-weekly exercise program. It consisted of swimming, basketball, volleyball, and calisthenics. Follow-up studies on these patients indicated a death rate of less than one-half the expected rate. Since the study was not carefully controlled (random assignment to exercise and nonexercise groups), the statistics are less meaningful.

In Canada, seventy-seven coronary patients in an exercise group were compared to a nonexercise group of 111 men of similar age and severity of heart disease. A seven-year follow-up revealed that 28 percent of the nonexercise group experienced recurrences (nonfatal) of heart attacks. The figure was only 1.3 percent in the exercise group. Twelve percent of the nonexercise group suffered cardiac deaths, which was three times that of the exercise group. A possible weakness in the study, however, was that the groups were not carefully screened for important risk factors such as cigarette smoking, blood pressure, and blood cholesterol levels.

One of the best designed studies comparing exercise and nonexercise coronary patients was reported from Finland. In this study, patients were assigned, at random, to exercise and control groups.

Unlike the Canadian study, the groups were similar with respect to age, smoking habits, blood cholesterol levels, and previous levels of physical activity. After an observation period of two years, there were no differences between the groups as to recurrences of heart attacks or deaths from coronary attacks. However, regular attendance was very poor in the exercise group and a significant number of the controls participated in exercise activities on their own. Therefore, it is not too surprising that group differences weren't detected.

Summary

The trend of almost all the epidemiological studies to date supports the theory that physical activity and regular exercise are of importance in both the prevention and treatment of coronary heart disease. Although many of these studies had certain flaws, it appears that both ongoing and future studies will be devoid of these weaknesses. Hopefully they may enable the medical community to state unequivocally whether or not physical inactivity is a major risk factor. Until these data become available and in view of the favorable trend in multiple existing studies, it would seem more than prudent to encourage regular physical activity on a national level.

Testing under exercise stress

There are certain limits to evaluating the condition of the heart in a resting state. One can have almost total blockage of the three major coronary arteries and still have a normal-sounding heart when the doctor examines it with his stethoscope. The patient whose coronary blockage is diagrammed in Figure 4–1 represents such an example. In a recent study, 16 percent of patients with severe blockage of all three major coronary arteries had normal electrocardiograms (ECG) and 29 percent of those with severe disease of two coronary vessels had similar findings. A doctor cannot make a complete assessment of the heart when examination is limited to the resting state. For that matter, neither can a professional coach assess the capability of a rookie quarterback by merely observing him sitting on the

Figure 4–1. Blockage of coronary arteries, but normal-sounding heart to doctor's stethoscope.

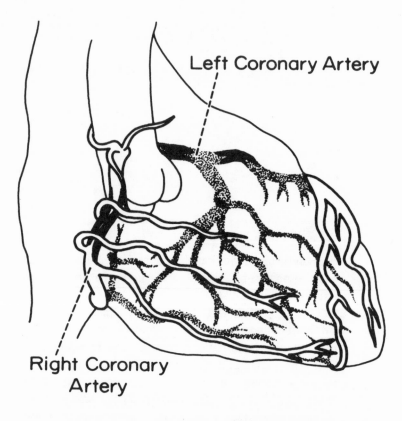

Left Coronary Artery

Right Coronary Artery

bench. The quarterback, and the heart, must be observed in action. For this reason, testing the heart under the stress of exercise has achieved increasing popularity. Certain historical aspects of such testing will be considered before discussing the methods and results of the technique.

Historical aspects

In 1928, only fourteen years after Paul Dudley White brought an electrocardiogram apparatus to this country from Europe, cardiologists described certain changes on the electrocardiogram *after* exercise in patients with coronary disease. The following year, another cardiologist described a simple tolerance test for circulatory efficiency, paving the way for future studies and advances in the field of exercise testing.

While some regard the treadmill as a modern exercise device, rather complex types were available in the early 1800s, thanks to a civil engineer named William Cubitt. In view of overcrowded prison conditions, it was difficult to find enough tasks so that hard labor sentences could be carried out. Cubitt solved the problem by devising different types of treadmills, one of which could employ 362 men simultaneously. Prison reformers, however, soon became less than enthusiastic about the device, charging that it produced exhaustion and emaciation. One stated that "the treadmill is, in reality, a species of torture, intruding itself under the semblance of labor." These same sentiments have probably been echoed more than once by patients who have undergone maximal treadmill stress testing in modern times.

Methods of testing

Although the treadmill is only one of several instruments used in exercise testing today, its popularity is increasing. The bicycle, which also

Figure 4–2 Treadmill testing with collection of expired air.

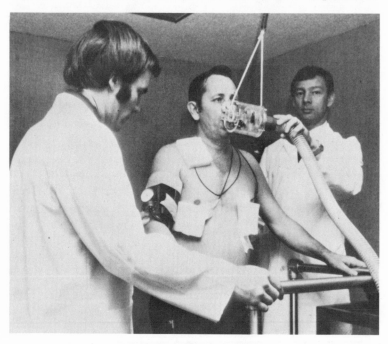

permits testing at various levels (or stages) of work, has been less popular in America than in Europe, owing to the fact that Americans are less accustomed to using their legs and experience greater lower extremity fatigue during testing.

The reasons for performing the exercise test are as follows:

1. It can be used as a diagnostic tool, looking for the electrocardiographic signs of insufficient blood supply to heart muscle or electrical instability of the heart that may indicate underlying coronary disease.

2. The exercise test can be used as an extension of the history and physical examination, permitting the physician to personally observe and assess exercise-induced symptoms ranging from chest pain to palpitations.

3. It can be used in a prognostic sense, usually in conjunction with other coronary factors, in a rough attempt at predicting the future risk of a coronary event.

4. Exercise testing can be used to measure one's level of cardiopulmonary fitness precisely, either directly by a simultaneous measurement of oxygen intake or indirectly by predicting the oxygen intake from the duration of the exercise.

One method of exercise testing involves ascending and descending two wooden steps a variable number of times (based on age and sex) for a three-minute period. While this test, named after Dr. Arthur Master, is the simplest and cheapest form of exercise testing, it has several limitations. The three-minute exercise period may be too strenuous for some, with pulse rates reaching as high as 190 beats per minute, and not strenuous enough for others. Another limitation is that the electrical activity of the heart is measured on the electrocardiogram only upon completion of the test and not during the actual period of exercise itself. Hence, the physician can miss important electrical events that occur only during exercise.

The treadmill device has achieved great popularity in recent years. Generally, the speed and slope of the motor-driven treadmill are increased at three-minute intervals. The electrocardiogram is recorded during and after exercise, and the test can be promptly terminated if the heart rate becomes too rapid.

Over an eighteen-month period, 250 persons underwent treadmill testing at Georgia Baptist Hospital. Eleven percent had abnormal tests indicative of inadequate blood supply to heart muscle and 21 percent had a variety of exercise-related heart rhythm disturbances.

The target heart rate to which a patient is exercised depends upon the clinical circumstances. Apparently healthy persons are exercised until their pulse rate exceeds 85 percent of the maximum rate for a particular age group, provided that they do not wish to stop sooner for various symptoms such as extreme fatigue. We use more caution in exercising patients with prior heart attacks, usually stopping the test when the heart rate exceeds 150 beats per minute.

Ischemia is the condition where insufficient blood is supplied to the heart muscle. The most widely accepted criterion for a "positive" exercise test for this condition is an ST segment depression of at least 1.0 mm that persists in a horizontal or downward slope for at least 0.08 seconds (Figure 4–3). An ST segment elevation of at least 1.0 mm is also considered to be indicative of a positive test, although experience with the latter is only a shadow of the former. When lower criteria are used (such as 0.5 mm of ST segment depression), the test becomes much less reliable in reflecting the presence or absence of underlying coronary disease. There are various factors that may cause spurious exercise electrocardiogram readings, such as drugs and glucose

Figure 4–3

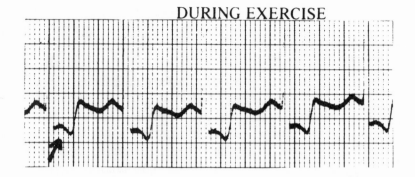

ingestion prior to the test. Such factors need to be identified in order to avoid overinterpretation of the results.

Predictive value

How reliable is the exercise stress test in predicting future coronary attacks? Several large groups of normal men have undergone exercise stress tests and have been observed for periods of up to ten years thereafter. In one such series of 756 middle-aged executives, the yield of abnormal stress tests was 3 percent. However, 70 percent of those in the latter group experienced the onset of coronary disease during the follow-up period. In other series, the yield of abnormal tests in otherwise healthy individuals ranged from 3 to 10 percent. Of these abnormal responders 30 to 70 percent developed symptoms of coronary disease within the next two and a half to ten years. Persons who had more markedly abnormal Master 2-step exercise tests had a coronary death rate fifteen times greater than those with normal tests over a ten-year period of observation.

Coronary arteriograms

Over 1000 men have undergone both exercise stress testing and coronary arteriography. Arteriography, the insertion of a catheter in a coronary artery, injecting dye, and filming the heart at work, is the most precise means available today of assessing coronary disease. Given one hundred patients with abnormal coronary arteriograms (i.e., greater than 50 percent occlusion of one of the three major coronary vessels), 75 percent will also have an abnormal treadmill stress test. Hence, the treadmill will miss 25 percent of those with significant coronary disease. On the other hand, given one hundred persons with normal coronary arteriograms, the treadmill test will be positive in 10 percent. Thus, it gives a false positive result in one out of every ten normal persons.

The Master 2-step test is even less reliable, missing 32 percent of those with coronary disease by arteriography and giving a false positive reading in 21 percent of those with normal coronary arteriograms. There are obviously significant limitations to exercise stress testing, and for this reason investigators are continuously trying to refine the test. On the other hand, when compared to coronary arteriography, exercise stress testing is considerably safer and less costly. It is also a noninvasive test, meaning that one does not have to make incisions in the skin or in the blood vessels themselves to carry out the procedure.

Summary

A brief review of exercise stress testing has included various methods and specific reasons for using the tests. Exercise stress testing has a certain value in predicting the risk of future coronary episodes. It would appear that the test plays an important role in our battle against coronary heart disease. Despite obvious limitations, it remains a safe, simple, and relatively inexpensive way to determine one's level of physical fitness and to detect subtle tendencies toward coronary disease.

5

How exercise
helps

Studies conducted on several species of animals indicate that the heart enlarges in response to chronic exercise. Wild animals, for instance, have larger hearts than do the more confined domestic animals. Hearts that are enlarged through exercise function normally, unlike hearts that become enlarged because of heart valve malfunctions or other diseased states.

Exercise appears to enhance the development of both the large and the small coronary arteries, which provide blood and oxygen to the working heart muscle. Wild rats and rabbits have a much greater network of small blood vessels throughout the heart than do their domestic counterparts. Age seems to be important in that exercise does not develop the small coronary vessel supply in older animals to the extent that it does in younger ones. Exercise seems to enhance the coronary circulation, and may provide alternate routes or detours for blood to flow in the event of a sudden blockage of a coronary artery. In an often quoted study, Dr. Richard Eckstein of Case Western Reserve University purposely narrowed the large coronary arteries of one hundred dogs and then divided those who developed heart attacks into two groups. He placed the dogs in the first group on a treadmill for five hours of exercise per week, while the dogs in the second group were kept in small cages over the two-month study. The coronary collateral blood vessels developed to a greater extent in the exercised dogs.

The efficiency of the heart also seems to be improved after exercise training. Exercised rats, when compared to nonexercised rats, were able to perform greater amounts of cardiac work and to pump more blood per minute. When the heart rates in both groups of rats were artificially increased by electrical stimulation (pacing) of the heart, the hearts of the physically trained rats were able to take in more oxygen.

Exercise also has a beneficial effect on the power generators (mitochondria) of skeletal and heart muscle. These power generators may show increases in both size and number.

Exercise may also affect blood cholesterol levels and the amount of atherosclerotic deposits in the blood vessel walls. Aleksandr Myasnikov, the late Russian heart specialist, placed a group of rabbits on a high cholesterol diet, exercising some and keeping others at rest. The exercised rabbits had lower blood cholesterol levels and less coronary atherosclerosis than the inactive rabbits. Physically active roosters showed a similar response (lower cholesterol and less atherosclerosis) although mongrel dogs behaved in an opposite fashion when exercised.

Exercise and risk factors

One of the ways by which physical activity might prevent or postpone the occurrence of coronary disease in man includes its effect on the various coronary risk factors. These effects are summarized below.

Serum cholesterol

Active physical conditioning programs have resulted in decreases in serum cholesterol levels in prisoners, army officers, postcoronary patients, and the general population. Nine blind men were exercised for only thirty-six minutes per week and decreased their cholesterol levels over a fifteen-week period. This reduction was independent of weight change. On the other hand, 101 military trainees did not show significantly decreased cholesterol levels despite sixteen hours per day of rugged basic training at boot camp. Several studies comparing college athletes and cross-country skiers with age-matched nonathletes showed no difference in cholesterol levels.

Serum triglyceride

While the effect of exercise on cholesterol levels is uncertain, most studies dealing with serum triglycerides suggest that exercise has a lowering effect, at least for a forty-eight-hour period. This might serve as an indication for the frequency of exercise sessions —every two days, at least.

High blood pressure

There are considerable data to suggest that exercise has only a modest effect in lowering the blood pressure of normal individuals and postcoronary patients. European cross-country skiers had an average systolic blood pressure lower than that of a nonactive group of similar age. Researchers showed that exercise resulted in an average drop of 13.5 mm Hg in the systolic blood pressure of hypertensive persons and a 12 mm Hg fall in the diastolic blood pressure. Those whose initial blood pressures fell within normal range had a decrease of 6 mm Hg in the diastolic blood pressure, but did not demonstrate a significant decrease in the systolic blood pressure.

Diabetes

Clinical experience indicates that persons with diabetes require less insulin when they are more physically active. Several reports have shown improvement of glucose tolerance and reductions of blood sugar levels after physical training. Whether such changes make the diabetic less susceptible to coronary disease is not known, however.

Overweight

Multiple studies show that significant weight

loss occurs in both normal and obese persons during prolonged physical exercise. Dr. Herman Hellerstein recorded an average weight reduction of five pounds in 158 men who exercised regularly for thirty-three months. Dr. Jean Mayer, a noted nutritional expert, has commented that the reason many people are obese is not always because they eat more, but because they exercise less than other people. Studies at the Mayo Clinic also indicate that one does not necessarily have to overeat to become fat, for as one ages, the basal metabolic requirements of the body tissues decrease. If exercise habits remain the same or decrease in frequency, obesity can develop even if there is some reduction of food intake.

Personality and behavior patterns

Cardiac patients who participate in exercise programs often show improvement in the depression and anxiety scales on the Minnesota Multiphasic Personality Inventory, a common psychological test consisting of 544 true-false questions. A group of fourteen college students was deprived of exercise during a thirty-day period, and as a consequence, displayed an increase in sexual tension and in anxiety, along with alterations in sleep patterns. The effects of physical training on personality traits of sixty middle-aged Purdue University faculty members were assessed, using the Cattell 16 Personality Factor Questionnaire. The high fitness group were more imaginative, self-sufficient, emotionally mature, and confident of conquering a certain goal than the less highly trained or untrained faculty members.

Miscellaneous effects of exercise

Although unaccustomed strenuous exercise can accelerate the processes of blood clotting and thrombus formation—clot formation in arteries—regular exercise tends to have the opposite effect. Since thrombus formation is felt by many to be an important precipitating event in a heart attack, this would appear to be an important effect of exercise. However, more studies are necessary before conclusions can be made in this area.

Other purported beneficial effects of exercise include a decrease in the stickiness of blood platelets (which may decrease the tendency for clot formation in arteries), a decrease in the adrenalin response to stress, and an enhancement of coronary collateral blood vessels. A study at the Mayo Clinic (in which the author participated) did not show any significant change in the latter after a year of physical training in ten patients with coronary disease, nor did a similar study in St. Petersburg, Florida.

Exercise might decrease the vulnerability of the heart to potentially serious rhythm disorders, such as spasmodic ventricular contractions. These probably account for most of the instances of instantaneous sudden deaths in this country. Heart specialists in Cleveland and in Minnesota have shown disappearance or lessening of erratic heart beats after an exercise training regimen. Since such erratic heart beats may subside spontaneously, and since multiple factors can be operational, it is difficult to say with certainty that physical training alone was therapeutic.

Summary

Exercise training appears to have a beneficial effect on body weight, blood pressure levels, blood sugar and serum triglyceride levels, and may also influence several psychosocial indices. Results on blood cholesterol levels are conflicting. Exercise improves the coronary collateral blood supply in many animals, but the effect in man has not been clearly demonstrated. The few studies available pertaining to the effect of physical training on blood clotting and on heart rhythm disturbances show largely beneficial influences.

6

Risks and precautions

Both physician and patient alike need to take certain precautions when involved in exercise stress testing or physical training. It does little good to detect a cardiac abnormality during an exercise test if it precipitates a coronary attack or a rhythm disturbance. If physical fitness programs are to succeed, the risks must be minimized. Newspapers have reported more than a few deaths among joggers. Death, no doubt, comes about when a person with multiple coronary risk factors suddenly tries to get in shape overnight, after spending thirty years or more growing out of shape. This chapter will deal with general guidelines for persons who are interested in having an exercise stress test and for those who want to initiate a physical training program.

For a normal individual the chances of dying

during or immediately following an exercise stress test are one in 10,000. For coronary patients or for persons with multiple coronary risk factors, chances are undoubtedly much higher. Risk can be minimized if certain precautions are taken.

First, the individual should never undergo stress testing if there is strong suspicion of a recent coronary episode (either a possible heart attack or a change in preexisting chest pain) or if the person does not feel well for any reason.

Second, emergency resuscitation equipment, including an electrical defibrillator, must always be immediately available. Medical personnel supervising the test should be thoroughly familiar with the equipment and make sure the defibrillator is fully charged before each day of testing. Monthly drills in the procedure of cardiac resuscitation are highly recommended. Third, the electrocardiogram must be closely watched during the test and the stress procedure should be terminated abruptly if there are disturbances in heart rhythm such as three or more consecutive premature beats. Fourth, the blood pressure should be closely followed during the recovery phase and the legs should be elevated in the recumbent position if the blood pressure falls below a systolic reading of 100 mm Hg. Fifth, the patient should be closely observed for a fifteen-to-twenty-minute period after the exercise test. He should be advised against taking a hot shower. The washroom should not be locked from the inside in the event of a sudden collapse while in the shower area.

To summarize, the person interested in undergoing an exercise stress test should do so only in a reputable medical laboratory under the direction of a physician. The test should be postponed in the event of a recent illness. If the person undergoing testing feels weak or lightheaded during the procedure, the physician should be signaled so that the test can be promptly terminated.

Physical fitness programs

The best way to enhance the safety of physical training programs is to make sure that individuals are properly screened and evaluated prior to starting such a program and to supervise them closely while they are progressively increasing their level of physical activity. Prior to commencing any physical conditioning program, it is absolutely essential that certain medical requirements be met. The apparently healthy person under age thirty needs only to have a complete medical history and physical examination within the preceding year. For those between ages thirty and forty, the examination should be done within three months of the starting date and should include a resting electrocardiogram (and preferably an exercise stress test). Those between the ages of forty-one and fifty-nine should definitely have an exercise stress test in addition to the medical examination. For the apparently healthy person over age fifty-nine, the physical examination needs to be done within two weeks of starting the fitness program and should include a resting and an exercise electrocardiogram. The person with known coronary heart disease should be at least two to three months post–heart attack before starting a long-range physical conditioning program. If such a program is limited to walking, it can be performed without medical supervision, provided a screening examination does not detect heart failure or serious disturbances in cardiac rhythm.

Postcoronary patients who wish to undergo more strenuous forms of conditioning, including jogging, and who do not have certain absolute contraindications to exercise should do so under the direct supervision of medical personnel and in the presence of emergency resuscitation equipment. Exclusions from the latter programs include persons with any of the following: 1) moderate to severe narrowing of the aortic heart valve, 2) heart failure, 3) a recent severe infectious disease, 4) severe exertion-induced chest pain, 5) inflammation of the veins, 6) serious heart rhythm disturbances, 7) poorly controlled blood pressure levels (systolic blood pressure more than 200 mm Hg, diastolic pressure more than 120 mm Hg), 8) weaknesses (aneurysms) in the wall of the aorta, and 9) certain types of cardiac pacemakers.

The following case history illustrates the necessity of a thorough medical evaluation:

A forty-year-old insurance salesman was hospitalized after complaining of severe chest pain that had developed while he was jogging in a Run For Your Life exercise class. He had previously been well, although he had not actively exercised in over twenty years. He had smoked two packs of cigarettes per day, had been moderately overweight all his adult life, and recently had consumed between three and six ounces of alcoholic beverages (a moderate to heavy level of consumption) per day. His father died from a heart attack at forty-two. Prior to entering the exercise program, the patient obtained the recommended blood pressure, pulse rate, and cholesterol level information from his private physician. An electrocardiogram was not taken. After three weeks of the calisthenics and jogging program, he had not lost his initial leg muscle soreness. While attempting to jog one and a half miles, he was unable to keep up with the others in his group. Finally, he alternated walking and jogging, fifty steps each, and then jogged almost one mile, after which he noted severe crushing chest pains associated with shortness of breath and sweating. On physical examination, his blood pressure was normal. Subsequent electrocardiograms showed evidence of a recent heart attack (myocardial infarction). The patient was discharged from the hospital at the end of the third week.

It is obvious that this individual was neither properly screened prior to the exercise program nor was he properly supervised during the early phase. It is fortunate that he survived the heart attack, for others have not been as lucky.

Dr. Meyer Friedman and collegues in San Francisco caution that instantaneous deaths in persons with severe coronary occlusion are not infrequent following strenuous physical activity. The cause of death is almost certainly a sudden disturbance in heart rhythm. Many persons who fall in this high-risk category can be properly identified through exercise stress testing.

In four years of exercise testing and supervising

physical training programs at Georgia Baptist Hospital, we have had two serious incidents, one occurring on the treadmill and one at the gymnasium. Both involved the abrupt onset of the potentially catastrophic rhythm disturbance, ventricular fibrillation. Thanks to the immediate availability of emergency equipment and of a well-organized medical team, both patients survived the episode and returned to the exercise program.

Exercise by prescription: The MET unit system

Few people know what constitutes proper physical exercise. Rather startling data were brought out by a research survey conducted in 1974 by the President's Council on Physical Fitness and Sports (PCPFS). For instance, as mentioned earlier, approximately 45 percent of adult Americans do not participate in any form of exercise; yet 57 percent of the adults sampled (49 million) felt that they were getting more than enough physical exercise. Oddly enough, nearly two-thirds of the nonexercisers actually felt that they were as physically fit as they ought to be.

Of the sixty million adults who said they did exercise, the more popular activities were as follows:

Walking	44.0 million
Bicycling	18.0
Swimming	14.0
Calisthenics	14.0
Jogging	6.5

While more than half of the walkers tended to do so on an almost daily basis, few who said they did other forms of exercise did them with any degree of regularity (i.e., three times per week).

The survey also revealed the types of group sports American adults prefer:

Bowling	20.0 percent
Swimming	18.0
Golf	9.0
Softball	8.5
Tennis	6.0
Volleyball	5.0
Water skiing	3.0
Snow skiing	2.0

Once again, it was rare to find those who performed the given sport at least three times per week.

Who is to blame for the rather pitiful state of our country's physical fitness? While the survey did not provide a direct answer to this question, it did indicate that 80 percent of those questioned had never been advised by their physicians to participate in regular physical activity. Of those who were told to exercise, most were advised to do so for a specific reason, such as recent abdominal surgery, an injured extremity, and the like. Even when the physician did state that a patient should "get a little exercise," he rarely indicated the type, frequency, intensity, or duration.

Exercise needs to be prescribed for a person, just as one receives a prescription for a certain drug. Patient response to a prescription for more exercise or for a drug needs to be precisely measured. One should also be made aware of certain side effects of both.

Physical fitness has several components, and these components can be remembered by the appropriate acronym—SAFE. S = strength; A = ability (skill) ; F = flexibility; E = endurance.

Exercise gimmicks come and go, promising instant fitness in three easy lessons. The isometric exercise craze is an example of an attempted shortcut to physical fitness. Although there is some laboratory evidence that pushing or pulling against walls or other stationary objects can indeed improve one's muscle strength in relatively brief sessions, there is little if any evidence to suggest that it improves heart and lung endurance. There is no evidence that the function of the cardiovascular and respiratory centers can be improved by pushing against an immovable object for six seconds per day.

This chapter deals with a system of accomplishing two important components of fitness—endurance and flexibility training. Ability and skill are largely achieved by constant practice, proper instructions, and innate talent. The development of enhanced strength, though of considerable importance to the athlete, is of much less importance to the coronary-prone American, and hence is omitted.

Endurance exercises

Dr. Kenneth Cooper made a significant contribution to the method of exercise prescription with a point system in the popular book, *Aerobics*. Dr. Cooper recommends that adults earn at least thirty points of exercise per week. One way to ac-

complish this is by jogging a mile in eight minutes
(this activity is worth five points), six days a week.
Recently, Dr. B. Grunewald came up with a similar
point system in the German publication *Die Gesund-
heits Karriere.*

Such point systems are rather arbitrary and
difficult to adapt for the coronary-prone person. In
view of this, the following point system has been
devised, based on sound physiological principles and
tailored to the individual. The system can even be
used by a postcoronary patient, provided that it is
done under medical supervision.

*Method of endurance exercise prescription
(the MET unit system)*

When considering endurance exercises to benefit the heart and lungs, it is important also to consider the pulse rate. Each person has a maximum
pulse rate, based on his or her age and degree of
physical conditioning. This rate can be predicted
from Table 7–1, or, more precisely, can be actually
measured by exercise stress testing.

Table 7–1

	Predicted heart rates (beats per minute)		
Age	*Maximal*	*85% Maximal*	*70% Maximal*
20	200	170	140
30	190	162	133
40	180	153	126
50	170	145	119
60	160	136	112
70	150	128	105

Exercise physiologists have found that one needs to perform exercises that will maintain the pulse rate at a level of at least 70 percent of the maximum rate for at least thirty-five to sixty minutes per week, preferably more than ninety minutes per week. The average housewife thinks she's in pretty good physical condition because she is relatively active much of the day. However, the activity is usually low-level and the pulse rate does not approach the 70 percent mark. When tested on a treadmill or bicycle ergometer, the housewife's level of fitness is often rather poor. The same can be said for a mailman, who walks a good deal but, again, infrequently achieves a maximum pulse rate level during the course of his day.

An exercise stress test is an absolute prerequisite before embarking on a physical fitness program. The maximum tolerance for physical work, and hence the maximum pulse rate, is measured. The pulse rate is converted into MET (or metabolic) units, and an exercise prescription is filled out, utilizing activities that constitute at least 70 percent of the maximum MET unit number. One MET unit is the amount of caloric energy a person expends in a resting state. In other words, it is the number of calories needed to maintain basic bodily functions. Five MET units, for example, is the amount of energy expenditure needed to walk at a rate of four miles per hour. Hence, this activity requires five times as much energy as does resting or sleeping.

If the level of maximal exercise on the treadmill is ten METS, 70 percent of this figure, or seven MET units, is selected as the intensity level for physical training. A list of activities recommended for this work level would include jogging (5 mph pace), bicycling (12 mph pace), swimming (side-stroke, 1 mph pace), home treadmill walking (3 mph, ten percent grade), and bench stepping (24 steps per minute, 35 cm step elevation). Mountain hiking (without a backpack) could be substituted for any of the above, as could activities like half-court basketball and touch football. In order to achieve adherence and to make the regimen more enjoyable, one must be able to choose among a variety of activities. It is this same variety that has been one of the strongest features of the *Aerobics* program. A list of endurance activities falling within various MET unit levels can be seen in Table 7-2.

Table 7-2 Endurance activities falling within various MET levels.

3-4 METS	Ping Pong
Badminton (doubles)	Raking leaves
Cycling (6 mph)	Rowing (noncompetitive)
Dancing (moderate)	Step-up (24 steps/minute,
Golf (pulling cart)	18 cm height)
Pitching horseshoes	Tennis (doubles)
Softball (excluding pitcher)	Treadmill (2 mph, 7% grade)
Steps (24 steps/minute,	
12 cm height)	*5-6 METS*
Treadmill (2 mph, 3.5% grade)	Cycling (10 mph)
Volleyball (6-man,	Horseback riding (trot)
not vigorous)	Ice skating
Walking (3 mph)	Roller skating
	Step-up (24 steps/minute,
4-5 METS	25 cm height)
Calisthenics (in general)	Swimming (1 mph)
Cycling (8 mph)	Treadmill (2 mph,
Dancing (vigorous)	10.5% grade)
Golf (carrying clubs)	Walking (4 mph)

Table 7–2 continued

6–7 METS	*8–9 METS*
Badminton (competition)	Basketball (vigorous)
Cycling (11 mph)	Cycling (13 mph)
Lawn-mowing (hand mower)	Fencing
Skiing (towing or easy downhill)	Handball
Square dancing	Jogging (5½ mph)
Step-up (24 steps/minute, 32 cm height)	Paddleball
Swimming (1.6 mph)	Step-up (30 steps/minute, 28 cm height)
Tennis (singles)	
Walking (5 mph)	*10–11 METS*
Water skiing	Handball (vigorous)
	Paddleball (vigorous)
7–8 METS	Running (6 mph)
Basketball (moderate)	Step-up (30 steps/minute, 36 cm height)
Cycling (12 mph)	Swimming (back stroke, 1.6 mph)
Horseback riding (gallop)	Treadmill (3.4 mph, 14% grade)
Jogging (5 mph)	
Mountain hiking (without back pack)	*12+ METS*
Skiing (hard, downhill)	Rowing (11 mph) 13½ METS
Step-up (24 steps/minute, 35 cm height)	Running (8 mph) 13½ METS
Swimming (side stroke, 1 mph)	Step-up (30 steps/minute, 40 cm height) 12 METS
Touch football	Treadmill (3.4 mph, 18% grade) 12 METS
Treadmill (3 mph, 10% grade)	

So far we have mainly considered the intensity of exercise. As previously alluded to, proper exercise training must also be of sufficient duration, preferably ninety minutes per week. If one divides the number of minutes by ten and multiplies this number by the MET unit prescription number, a scoring system is arrived at which considers both intensity and duration of exercise. Let's see how this works out for a given normal executive.

Fred, a forty-year-old banker, completed the fourth stage of the Bruce treadmill test (in which the treadmill speed and slope increase at three-minute intervals). This stage is equivalent to 13 MET units, which is his maximal tolerance for physical work (and which raised his pulse rate to 187 beats per minute). His exercise prescription would call for activities equivalent to 70 percent of thirteen MET units or nine METs. Handball, paddleball, and basketball are sports which fall in this caloric expenditure level. The nine MET units of activity should be performed for ninety minutes per week. By dividing the number of minutes by ten, the number of exercise minutes is nine; one then multiplies those nine METs, so the exercise prescription would call for 81 units per week. A daily (or weekly) scorecard could be kept. For instance, if Fred performs step-up exercises at the nine MET level (thirty steps per minute, twenty-eight cm height) for ten minutes on one day, he will earn nine times 10/10 or nine units. If he plays twenty minutes of handball the next day, he will earn nine (METS) times 20/10 or eighteen units.

To summarize, the prescription of endurance exercise by using the MET unit system can be performed by the following approach:

> *Step 1*—Determine the maximum tolerance of physical work on the treadmill or bicycle ergometer and convert to MET units.

> *Step 2*—Calculate the training level of MET units (70 percent of the maximum MET tolerance).
>
> *Step 3*—Divide the weekly number of desired minutes (90) of endurance exercise by 10.
>
> *Step 4*—Multiply the above times the training level of MET units.
>
> *Step 5*—The product of Step 4 becomes the weekly exercise unit system goal.

The untrained normal individual must start slowly for the first few weeks of exercise to avoid undue muscular strain. A suggested endurance exercise schedule for a beginner in below-average condition is as follows:

Week	Duration (minutes)	Frequency/week
1–2	15 (at the prescribed MET unit level)	3 times
3–4	15	4
5–6	15	5
7–8	15	6

Beginning at week nine, one can select one of the training schedules below, adapting it to personal preference and to the leisure time available for exercise:

	Minutes	Times per week
1)	13	7
2)	15	6
3)	18	5
4)	22½	4
5)	30	3

The author has a maximal treadmill tolerance of fourteen METS and trains at 70 percent of this, or ten METS. The latter is accomplished by jogging at a speed of six mph. Because of hospital duties, the 22.5 minutes, four times per week schedule is preferred and the weekly unit earnings are 90 minutes/ 10 x 10 METS or 90 units.

It is advisable to record your exercising in a log book and review it periodically with a physician. For at least the first six to twelve months of an exercise program, one should undergo repeat exercise stress testing at three-month intervals to quantify the training effect and to adjust the exercise prescription (as the maximal level of physical work on the stress test increases).

It is often difficult to arrange one's work schedule so that it will coincide with a partner's. Therefore, one should be particularly aware of the endurance activities that can be done alone. These include: walking at a brisk pace; jogging; swimming; cycling; skipping rope; bench stepping (stepping up and down on a wooden bench); ice skating; cross-country skiing; canoeing; aerobic dancing to music.

Except for swimming and ice skating, none of these activities requires either a special facility or a certain amount of skill. These activities should constitute the majority of time spent in cardiopulmonary endurance activities. As previously mentioned, they can be supplemented by group activities (see Table 7–2). Participation will depend on the age and overall condition of the individual. Hockey would obviously not be prescribed for the average sixty-year-old. An additional advantage of individual activities is the ease with which they can be performed. For instance, the businessman who travels extensively could easily pack a jump rope or a pair of walking or jogging shoes. He might swim in a hotel pool or perhaps carry a collapsable stationary cycle in the trunk of his car. Easier still, he could measure the elevation of a certain object in his room, such as a chair or a stool, and use it for bench-stepping exercise. A minimum of time is required and the return is well worth the investment.

Endurance exercise for the coronary patient

The MET unit system can be used to prescribe endurance exercise for the postcoronary patient as well as the patient with multiple coronary risk factors. In such instances, the maximum tolerance for physical work on the treadmill will be a symptom-limited performance. The patient will have a lessened workload and often will stop much sooner because of symptoms like chest pain or severe shortness of breath. In that case, the training prescription (in METs) should be 70 percent of the symptom-limited maximum MET unit performance.

If the postcoronary patient cannot exercise under direct medical supervision, the above method should not be used. Rather, the endurance exercise should be limited to brisk walking, for safety reasons, and a specific walking regimen can be utilized depending upon the amount of time that has elapsed since the recent heart attack.

Table 7–3 is a home walking schedule for the uncomplicated (i.e., no heart failure, rhythm disturbance, etc.) postcoronary patient immediately upon returning home from the hospital. Table 7–4 is a suggested regimen to begin three months after a coronary episode. Neither should be undertaken without the knowledge and consent of one's personal physician.

Table 7–3 Exercise regimen
(one to twelve weeks after infarction).

Weeks	*Activity*
1–3	In-hospital exercise regimen.
4	Walk five minutes at leisurely pace (¼ mile) once per day.
5	Walk five minutes at leisurely pace (¼ mile) twice per day.
6	Walk ten minutes at leisurely pace (½ mile) once per day.
7	Walk ten minutes at leisurely pace (½ mile) once per day.
8	Walk fifteen minutes at leisurely pace (¾ mile) once per day.
9	Walk fifteen minutes at leisurely pace (¾ mile) once per day.
10	Walk twenty minutes at leisurely pace (1 mile) once per day.
11	Walk twenty minutes at moderate pace (1⅓ mile) once per day.
12	Walk thirty minutes at moderate pace (2 miles) once per day.
13	Begin group activity program.

Table 7–4 Home exercise program
(twelve weeks after infarction).

Weeks	*Activity*
1–2	Measure 1-mile distance with car. Walk to this point and back (total of 2 miles) in 40 minutes. Pulse at end should be less than 115 per minute.*

3–4   Measure 1.5-mile distance. Walk to this point and back (3 miles) in 60 minutes.

5–6   Measure 2-mile distance. Walk to this point and back (4 miles) in 72 minutes.

7–9   Measure 2-mile distance. Walk to this point and back (4 miles) in 60 minutes (15-minute mile pace).

10–12 Measure 2-mile distance. Walk to this point and back (4 miles) in 56 minutes (14-minute mile pace, just below a slow jog).

*The individual is taught to check his own pulse rate. He is not to advance to the next stage (as from weeks 1–2 to weeks 3–4) unless the immediate postexercise heart rate is less than 115 per minute.

For the postcoronary patient who is fortunate to live near a cardiac rehabilitation center, the walking activity can be supplemented with a jogging program in most instances. The walk-jog regimen which this writer initiated in conjunction with YMCA director Edward Koch at the Mayo Clinic in 1967 is given in Table 7–5. All patients must be referred to

Table 7–5 Medically supervised walk-jog regimen (twelve weeks after infarction).

Weeks	Activity
1–4	Walk slowly 100 yards, then briskly 100 yards, alternately for ¼ mile.
5–8	Walk slowly 100 yards, then briskly 100 yards, alternately for ½ mile.
9–12	Walk slowly 100 yards, walk briskly 100 yards, then jog 100 yards, alternately for ½ mile.
13–15	Walk briskly 200 yards, then jog 200 yards, alternately for ¾ mile.
16–24	Walk 200 yards, then jog 400 yards, alternately for 1 mile.
25–51	Jog 1 mile (maintain pulse rate at 70 percent maximal).
52 and over	Jog 2 miles.

the program by their private physician. Exercise stress-testing and/or patient interviews are conducted before advancing from one stage to the next. If a cardiac patient is having trouble, either in the form of chest pain or shortness of breath, his level of exercise is reduced, no matter how long he or she has been in the program. Patients are taught to check their own pulse rates before and after the walk-jog activity. Rates above 140 beats per minute are reported to the medical supervisor. The patients' skill and reliability in pulse rate recording is spot-checked by a nurse or physician. A nurse also queries the participants regarding the presence of chest pain within the prior forty-eight hour period. Any pain of greater than fifteen minutes' duration means that additional exercise must be stopped until the patient is seen by a physician.

This program has been employed at the Mayo Clinic ever since 1967. At Georgia Baptist Hospital in Atlanta, over 250 coronary patients have undergone exercise training by this technique. The effects of such a program have been similar to those described by Dr. Herman Hellerstein (Cleveland), Dr. Peter Rechnitzer (Canada) and Dr. Max Halhuber (Germany); namely, the beneficial effects include the ability to perform a given amount of physical work at a lower energy cost to the heart and the subjective psychological improvement that often occurs when one is no longer thought of as an invalid.

Prescribing flexibility exercises

There are many books which describe different calisthenic programs. At the Preventive Cardiology Clinic, we prefer a list of flexibility exercises which reach the major muscle groups. The exercises are divided into two groups, A and B (see figures at the end of this chapter). Group A exercises are a progressive schedule for normal persons (i.e., persons with no clinical evidence of coronary disease). Group B is a regimen for persons with multiple coronary risk factors or for patients with known coronary heart disease. Many of the exercises can be done to music, making it more enjoyable.

Summary

Few Americans are physically fit. Fewer still realize this seemingly obvious fact. Physicians are not taking an active role in prescribing exercise for their patients, and they often turn to expensive and essentially worthless exercise spas and exercise gimmicks.

It is not difficult for the general physician to prescribe exercise. Described was a five-step approach to the prescription of endurance exercise, based on the physiologically sound MET unit system, along with home-walking regimens for postcoronary patients. A second component of physical fitness, namely flexibility, was also described. Through the joint efforts of the general public and their physicians, 49 million Americans could profit through enhanced fitness and health.

Figure 7–1 Small jumps (the subject jumps approximately 4–6 inches vertically, landing on the anterior aspect of the feet).

	Repetitions	
Week	Level A	Level B
1–2	8	8
3–4	10	8
5–6	12	10
7–8	14	12
9–10	16	14
11–12	18	14
13–14	18	16
15–16	18	16
17–18	20	18
19–20	20	18
21–22	22	20
23–24	22	20

Figure 7–2 Arm circling (the arms are elevated in a horizontal position and rotated, first clockwise for the given number of repetitions, and then counterclockwise for the same number of times).

	Repetitions	
Week	Level A	Level B
1–2	6	4
3–4	6	4
5–6	8	4
7–8	8	6
9–10	10	6
11–12	10	6
13–14	10	8
15–16	10	8
17–18	12	8
19–20	12	10
21–22	14	10
23–24	14	10

Figure 7–3 Arm and shoulder loosening (with subject in standing position the arms are raised overhead, bringing palms together; the arms are then lowered to the sides, completing the sequence).

Week	Repetitions	
	Level A	*Level B*
1–2	6	6
3–4	8	6
5–6	10	8
7–8	12	8
9–10	14	10
11–12	14	10
13–14	14	12
15–16	16	12
17–18	16	12
19–20	18	14
21–22	18	14
23–24	20	16

Figure 7–4 Side twisters (the subject twists his trunk to the left, returns to the starting position, then twists to the right. Return to the starting position completes one cycle).

Week	Repetitions	
	Level A	*Level B*
1–2	6	4
3–4	8	5
5–6	10	6
7–8	10	8
9–10	12	10
11–12	12	12
13–14	12	12
15–16	12	12
17–18	14	12
19–20	14	14
21–22	14	14
23–24	14	14

Figure 7–5 Reach 'n stretch (subject raises arms overhead and raises up onto toes, returning to the starting position).

Week	Repetitions	
	Level A	*Level B*
1–2	6	4
3–4	8	4
5–6	10	6
7–8	10	6
9–10	12	6
11–12	12	6
13–14	12	8
15–16	12	8
17–18	14	8
19–20	14	10
21–22	16	10
23–24	16	10

Figure 7–6 Jumping jack (start with arms at sides and feet together. Legs move laterally as palms are touched overhead).

Week	Repetitions	
	Level A	*Level B*
1–2	4	omit
3–4	6	
5–6	8	
7–8	8	
9–10	10	
11–12	10	
13–14	10	
15–16	10	
17–18	12	
19–20	12	
21–22	14	
23–24	14	

Figure 7–7 Elbow-knee (with hands behind the head, subject attempts to touch right elbow to left knee, assumes the upright position, then touches left elbow to right knee).

	Repetitions	
Week	Level A	Level B
1–2	4	4
3–4	4	5
5–6	6	6
7–8	6	8
9–10	8	10
11–12	8	12
13–14	10	12
15–16	10	12
17–18	12	12
19–20	12	14
21–22	14	14
23–24	14	14

Figure 7–8 Lateral bend (subject bends laterally to the right, assumes an erect position, then bends laterally to the left).

	Repetitions	
Week	Level A	Level B
1–2	4	4
3–4	4	5
5–6	6	6
7–8	6	8
9–10	8	10
11–12	8	12
13–14	10	12
15–16	10	12
17–18	10	12
19–20	12	14
21–22	12	14
23–24	12	14

Figure 7–9   Neck rotation (head is rotated clockwise in a circular fashion, then counterclockwise—omit if any history of dizziness or lightheadedness).

| | Repetitions | |
Week	Level A	Level B
1–2	2	omit
3–4	2	
5–6	4	
7–8	4	
9–10	6	
11–12	6	
13–14	6	
15–16	6	
17–18	8	
19–20	8	
21–22	8	
23–24	8	

Figure 7–10   Leg crossover (while lying supine, subject raises the right leg and touches the floor on his left with his toes; after returning to a flat position, complete one cycle by touching left toes to the floor on the right).

| | Repetitions | |
Week	Level A	Level B
1–2	4	2
3–4	4	2
5–6	6	4
7–8	6	4
9–10	8	4
11–12	8	6
13–14	8	6
15–16	8	8
17–18	10	8
19–20	10	10
21–22	12	10
23–24	12	10

Figure 7-11   Rocking sit-ups (while lying supine with arms at sides, subject rocks to a sitting position and then returns to a supine position).

	Repetitions	
Week	*Level A*	*Level B*
1–2	4	2
3–4	4	4
5–6	6	4
7–8	6	4
9–10	8	6
11–12	8	6
13–14	10	6
15–16	10	8
17–18	12	8
19–20	12	8
21–22	14	10
23–24	14	10

Figure 7-12   Knee-chest (from a supine position, subject grasps the right knee and flexes the thigh: then repeat the maneuver with the left knee, completing one repetition).

	Repetitions	
Week	*Level A*	*Level B*
1–2	6	4
3–4	8	6
5–6	10	8
7–8	10	8
9–10	10	10
11–12	10	10
13–14	12	10
15–16	12	10
17–18	14	12
19–20	14	12
21–22	16	14
23–24	16	14

Figure 7–13 **Alternate straight-leg raising (while lying supine the subject elevates the left leg to a 45-degree angle with the floor, keeping the knee straight; repeat this with the right leg, completing one sequence).**

Week	Repetitions	
	Level A	Level B
1–2	4	2
3–4	6	3
5–6	8	4
7–8	8	6
9–10	10	8
11–12	10	10
13–14	12	10
15–16	12	10
17–18	14	12
19–20	14	12
21–22	16	14
23–24	16	14

Figure 7–14 **Pushups (subject positions himself on his hands and toes, touching chest to the floor; postcoronary patients are restricted to knee-pushups).**

Week	Repetitions	
	Level A	Level B
1–2	6	4
3–4	8	6
5–6	8	8
7–8	10	8
9–10	12	10
11–12	12	12
13–14	14	14
15–16	14	14
17–18	16	14
19–20	16	16
21–22	18	16
23–24	18	16

Figure 7–15 Scissors (subject assumes a sprinter's position with right leg forward and left leg back; the positions of the feet are reversed in a bouncing movement).

Week	Repetitions Level A	Level B
1–2	4	omit
3–4	4	
5–6	6	
7–8	6	
9–10	6	
11–12	8	
13–14	8	
15–16	8	
17–18	10	
19–20	10	
21–22	10	
23–24	10	

Figure 7–16 Chest-leg raise (assuming a prone position, the subject places the arms overhead and raises the upper part of the body and the legs as far off the ground as possible).

Week	Repetitions Level A	Level B
1–2	4	2
3–4	6	3
5–6	8	5
7–8	8	8
9–10	10	10
11–12	10	10
13–14	12	10
15–16	12	10
17–18	12	10
19–20	14	12
21–22	14	12
23–24	14	12

Figure 7–17 Side leg raise (with subject on right side, the left leg is elevated for the recommended number of repetitions; then switch to the left side and raise the right leg the same number of times).

Week	Repetitions Level A	Level B
1–2	6	4
3–4	8	6
5–6	10	8
7–8	10	8
9–10	10	10
11–12	12	10
13–14	12	10
15–16	14	10
17–18	14	12
19–20	14	12
21–22	16	14
23–24	16	14

Figure 7-18 Trunk twist (the subject sits with legs out straight and with arms raised to a horizontal position; twist the trunk to the left, return to the original position, and complete one sequence by twisting the trunk to the right).

Week	Repetitions Level A	Level B
1–2	6	4
3–4	8	6
5–6	10	8
7–8	10	8
9–10	10	10
11–12	12	10
13–14	12	12
15–16	14	12
17–18	14	12
19–20	14	14
21–22	16	14
23–24	16	14

Figure 7–19 **Reverse pushups (the subject assumes a sitting position with legs out straight and hands on the floor behind the back; he pushes his body off the floor and then returns to the original position).**

	Repetitions	
Week	*Level A*	*Level B*
1–2	4	2
3–4	4	3
5–6	6	4
7–8	6	5
9–10	8	6
11–12	8	6
13–14	10	8
15–16	10	8
17–18	10	8
19–20	12	10
21–22	12	10
23–24	12	10

Figure 7–20 **Reach 'n touch (the subject assumes a sitting position with legs slightly flexed and arms at the sides; he touches the toes with his fingertips and returns to the resting position).**

	Repetitions	
Week	*Level A*	*Level B*
1–2	6	4
3–4	8	6
5–6	8	8
7–8	10	8
9–10	10	10
11–12	12	10
13–14	12	12
15–16	14	12
17–18	14	12
19–20	14	14
21–22	14	14
23–24	14	14

8

Athletes' hearts: Diseased and nondiseased

A twenty-eight-year-old professional football player dies suddenly during a game and is found to have extensive atherosclerosis of the coronary arteries at autopsy. A relief pitcher experiences a heart attack but returns to the major leagues after a period of recovery and sets a record. A college football player has severe palpitations after sprinting. A professional athlete is traded to another team but fails the physical examination because of an abnormal electrocardiogram. A marathon runner cannot get life insurance because of an enlarged heart and a heart murmur. These are but a few examples of cardiac disease and nondisease that may be found in the athlete. Since one might develop a so-called athlete's heart through an exercise prescription such as described in Chapter 7, it is important that we learn something about this entity.

Historical aspects

Athlete's heart has been of concern to physicians ever since the time of Hippocrates. Deaths in young athletes have been lamented by poets and meticulously studied by pathologists. Until this century, most physicians felt that the condition known as athlete's heart was not conducive to optimal cardiac performance.

As previously noted, a leader in dispelling many of these misconceptions was the late Dr. Paul Dudley White, whose reports on the marathon runner, Clarence De Mar, and on former Harvard football lettermen indicated that lifelong participation in athletics might indeed be advantageous to the heart.

Cardiac nondisease

Clarence De Mar probably had one of the first cases of cardiac nondisease. After his first marathon race, he was found to have a heart murmur and did not compete in this event again for eight years.

Endurance athletes not infrequently have systolic heart murmurs. Forceful heart beats and very slow resting heart rates are common findings in well-trained athletes. Gaston Roelants, the great Belgian distance runner, reportedly had a resting heart rate of 38 beats per minute, as did author-runner Hal Higdon.

The athlete's chest X-ray may show cardiac enlargement, due to hypertrophy, an increase in size of heart muscle fibers. There is no evidence to date that an enlarged heart indicates abnormal heart performance. A number of variations on an athlete's electrocardiogram may be recorded that may resemble coronary heart disease. Indeed, when I show a copy of Wilt Chamberlain's electrocardiogram to medical residents, I am usually given a diagnosis of an impending heart attack.

Cardiac disease

The athlete is, of course, subject to disease of the heart that may have been present at birth (congenital) or acquired in early or later life. The occurrence of coronary artery atherosclerosis in the young football player who died on the field is not surprising in view of autopsy studies on young soldiers and young victims of auto accidents, most of whom showed evidence of the disease. Dietary indiscretions of football linemen and weight fluctuations in wrestlers may contribute to the premature hardening of the coronary arteries.

In contact sports, chest injuries can cause a variety of cardiac lesions including dysfunction of the heart valves and bruising of the heart muscle itself.

In several instances, sudden death in young athletes has been attributed to abnormalities of the heart rhythm, present since birth. Some of these heart rhythm disturbances may be hereditary. I recently experienced this in a seventeen-year-old boy who collapsed while playing football. His electrocardiogram showed abnormalities in rhythm that also appeared in electrocardiograms performed on four other family members.

Summary

The well-trained athlete may, on clinical and laboratory examination of the heart, have characteristics that mimic disease states. Physicians, trainers, and the athletes themselves should be aware of this occurrence so that a proper diagnosis of cardiac nondisease can be made.

At the same time, the athlete is subject to both congenital and acquired disease of the heart. Symptoms and signs of such diseases may first be detected under the stress of physical training or may eventually be discovered when a routine electrocardiogram is interpreted as abnormal.

Athletes with complaints of exercise-related palpitations, chest pain, and black-out spells should be carefully studied with electrocardiogram monitoring and exercise stress testing.

Since coronary atherosclerosis occurs in nearly epidemic proportions in this country and apparently begins early in life, thought should be given to the possibility of changing the dietary habits of amateur and professional athletes.

9

Fitness: Cases, characters, and customs

A physician cannot be active in athletics and in the research of physical fitness and fail to be impressed by the phenomenal capacity of the human organism for exercise and by the unique personalities and characteristics of athletes themselves.

The human being is capable of doing more than 14,000 consecutive sit-ups and 6,000 consecutive push-ups. Man can run almost thirteen miles in one hour or 121¼ miles nonstop. A thirty-four-year-old Australian, Tony Rafferty, recently ran 3,686 miles across the continent of Australia in seventy-four days, averaging nearly fifty miles per day. Bill Emmerton, whom I had the pleasure of meeting at the Boston Marathon, has run over 105,000 miles in his lifetime, including several jaunts of 125 miles or more in the 106° F. Death Valley heat. Walt Stack, sixty-one years young, placed sixth in a 100-mile race run in three segments over a three-day period. Not to be outdone, seventy-five-year-old Fred Grace competes in similar races by keeping up a training program that consists of running twenty to thirty miles on alternate days and lifting weights the other days for relaxation.

Cases

I have had the opportunity to evaluate two men who illustrate the human ability to become or remain in excellent physical condition despite advancing years.

Jon Robere, a youngster who recently turned sixty, plays the organ at the Read House in Chattanooga, Tennessee, at night and gives music lessons during the day. In between, he participates in distance races that include marathon events.

Jon was active in swimming, diving, and tumbling as a child, but didn't take up distance running until age fifty-four. Over a nine-month period, he gradually built up his jogging to one mile every day. He then became interested in long-distance racing and gradually increased his annual jogging mileage from 400 miles in 1955 to over 3000 miles in 1973. His best marathon time was three hours and thirty-two minutes. He was timed in forty-one minutes for the six-mile run and sixty-seven minutes for the ten-mile distance. He seldom runs the mile, but has been clocked at five minutes and fifty-eight seconds in that event.

Jon has an interesting family history in that his father lived to be ninety-five and his mother,

Figure 9–1   Jon Robere.

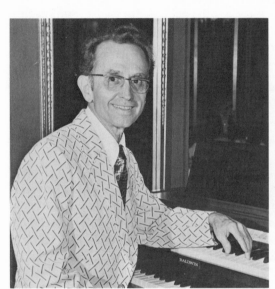
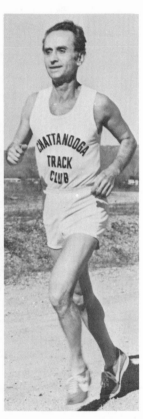

eighty-eight. He weighs 122 pounds, only 6 percent
of which is fat. His blood pressure is in the low
normal range and his resting pulse rate is fifty-five
beats per minute. Laboratory tests include a serum
cholesterol of 223 mg percent, well below average for
a man of his age. His serum triglyceride level was

extremely low at 45 mg percent. Jon completed thirteen minutes on the Bruce treadmill test. His maximum oxygen consumption of 42 ml/kg/min. was
very high for his age group. The exercise electrocardiogram did reveal some irregularities in cardiac
rhythm when the pulse rate rose above 150 beats
per minute. As a result, he was advised to maintain
his exercise pulse rate at least ten beats below this
level and to concentrate on long slow distance (LSD)
training rather than interval work.

Seventy-one-year-old Tom Roberts waited until
sixty to take up jogging. Prior to that, he had never
participated in athletics and his only form of leisure
activity consisted of sporadic yard work. Tom upped
his weekly jogging to twelve miles a week at sixty-
two, and four years later, responding to a suggestion
made in jest by a friend, he began to train for the
Boston Marathon. He participated in that event for
five consecutive years. In 1968, his time for the
Marathon was just over three and one-half hours,
earning 215th place. He was the oldest man to finish
the race.

His past medical history indicated that he had
been a mild cigarette smoker, but had quit over
thirty years ago. His five brothers and sisters have
all lived past the age of sixty-five and none has any
unusual athletic abilities.

On physical examination, Tom's blood pressure
was a healthy 130/80 mm Hg and the heart rate was
fifty-eight beats per minute. His total weight of 134
lbs. included only 9 percent body fat.

Exercise stress testing, again by the Bruce
treadmill method, indicated a duration of thirteen
and one-half minutes, a remarkable achievement con-

sidering his age. The maximum heart rate during exercise was 165 beats per minute and the maximum blood pressure was 180/75 mm Hg. His maximal oxygen consumption of 55 ml/kg/min. was the highest ever reported in this age group, far exceeding the highest level (40 ml/kg/min) recorded in three distance runners of the seventy to seventy-nine age group.

Several weeks after completing the exercise stress test, Tom participated in an AAU-sanctioned one-mile race. His time of 6:13 enabled him to eclipse Virgil Sturgill's world record of 6:55 which was set in 1969 (see Figure 9–2). When Harold Chapson

Figure 9–2 Tom Roberts (center) after his world-record one-mile run. Defending champion, Virgil Sturgill (age 76, on Tom's left), and Elmer Sanborn (on Tom's right, age 72).

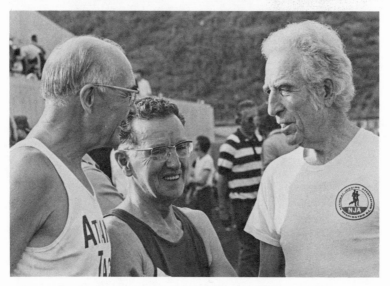

Courtesy Bud Skinner (*Atlanta Journal*)

subsequently lowered the mark to 6:04 at the 47th Rainbow Relays at the University of Hawaii, Tom responded by running 3,000 meters in 12:11:8, bettering the old record by over twenty-four seconds at the Tyler Cup race in Dallas.

Another case of great interest to me from the standpoint of rehabilitation involves John Hiller, the ace left-handed relief pitcher of the Detroit Tigers. Hiller suffered a heart attack in 1971. At that time he was overweight (220 lbs.), smoked two to three packs of cigarettes per day and was in poor physical condition. Following an initial recovery phase, during which he gave up the cigarettes, he lost weight, had an operation to decrease his intestinal absorption of dietary cholesterol and began jogging on a regular basis.

During the 1973 baseball season, the rehabilitation program paid off for John Hiller. He set a major league record for relief pitchers by saving thirty-six games. His earned run average was below 1.5 runs per game. It was only fitting that he should receive the annual Hutch award for his courageous comeback.

Characters

When it comes to characters, take sixty-five-year-old Johnny Kelley. Since 1927, Kelley has appeared in over 1,000 official races of one mile or longer and has completed ninety-three of ninety-six Marathon attempts. In so doing, he has become almost a legend at the annual Boston Marathon, winning it on two occasions and placing second seven times. His marathon time of 2:37:42 at age fifty-four is hard to believe. When he's not engaged in competition, Johnny is busy with his oil paintings in his art studio in East Dennis, Massachusetts.

Another character, who also happens to be a close family friend, is Dr. Joe Kopcha, an obstetrician from Gary, Indiana. Dr. Joe was a stalwart lineman on the great Chicago Bear football team of the 1930s. In addition to being an amateur actor, he operates a printing press in his basement, specializing in humorous cards. Throughout his life he has maintained a high level of physical fitness by playing tournament handball at least four to five times a week. Now in his late sixties and ten pounds lighter, Joe Kopcha looks fit enough to slip on the pads and terrorize opposing quarterbacks once again.

My favorite character has to be Larry Lewis, a former waiter at the St. Francis Hotel in San Francisco, who recently died at 106 of liver cancer. While working at the hotel, it was Larry's custom to walk five miles daily to and from work. As if this wasn't enough, Larry also added a six-mile daily jog and a vigorous swim. When he passed the century mark, Larry ran the 100-yard dash in seventeen seconds, claiming a world record for his age group.

While in San Francisco on business a year ago, I looked up Mr. Lewis. I found him in an office on Market Street, busily involved in his new job as goodwill ambassador for Western Girls, Inc., an employment agency. I was fascinated during our visit by hearing of his remarkable adventures. He grew up in the territory which became the city of Phoenix, Arizona. He claimed to have been taught the mysteries of health and well-being by an Indian chief called Ironshell, the same man who was one of

Figure 9–3 Dr. Joe Kopcha.

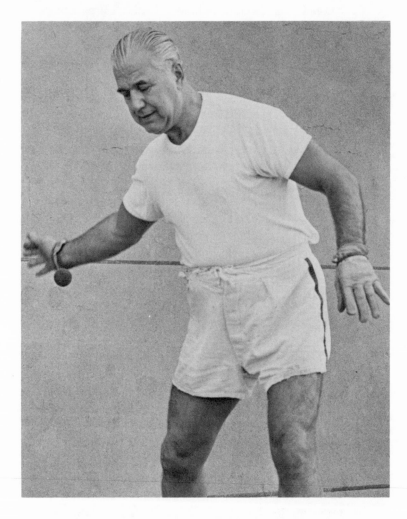

the models for the Indian on the old Indian-head nickel. Ironshell was no spring chicken himself, living to the ripe old age of 134. Larry told me how he used to work with Houdini until 1926, of how at 136 pounds, he was able to lift a man weighing twice that much, and how he habitually ate only natural foods and drank only purified water.

It would have been easy to question the man, to try to pick holes in his theories and to find flaws and inconsistencies in his stories. However, on the afternoon of our visit, during a period in which the credibility of our governmental leaders was at an all-time low, I preferred to believe this kindly man who was raised by the Indians and who continued their primitive customs of daily exercise and Spartan eating habits up until the time of his death.

Customs

The physical endurance and/or longevity of various isolated groups in the world, such as the Tarahumara Indians of Northern Mexico, the Masai tribesmen of East Africa, the Sherpa herdsmen of the Himalayan region, and the centenarians of Asia and South America have intrigued physicians and anthropologists for years.

Dr. Alexander Leaf, on sabbatical leave from Massachusetts General Hospital, traveled to Vilcabamba (in the Ecuadorean Andes), Hunza (Karakoren range of Kashmir), and Abkhazia (in the Caucasus mountain region of Russia). Dr. Leaf selected these people for careful scrutiny because of the high incidence of centenarians per 100,000 population. One finds only three centenarians per 100,000 people in the United States, but the figure is sixty-three per 100,000 in regions such as Abkhazia. After living with these people and observing their lifestyle,

Dr. Leaf surmised that low-calorie and low-fat diets, reduced levels of psychosocial stress, and high levels of physical conditioning were among the possible secrets for such unusual longevity. Most of the centenarians continued to work and to exercise regularly at elevations of up to 6,000 feet, indicative of highly efficient heart and lung function. Although he had trouble getting precise scientific data in the study, Dr. Leaf was apparently impressed with the effects of vigorous exercise on these people, and became a regular jogger himself when he returned to the Boston area.

The spectacular physical feats of the Tarahumara tribe in northern Mexico were described in the 1890s when the explorer, Carl Lumholtz, gave an account of their customs, including ultralong distance racing. These people were hunters and gatherers; their weapons were primitive. In hunting wild turkey and deer, the Indians would chase the animal, sometimes for several days, until it dropped from exhaustion. The long-distance races extended up to 150 miles and were made even more difficult by the mountainous terrain.

Coronary heart disease is virtually nonexistent in these people. Those who agreed to brief physical evaluations by several Oklahoma investigators were found to have low blood pressure readings, serum cholesterol levels that were often below 100 mg percent, and no evidence of heart enlargement or of heart disease. Interestingly, the main factor limiting the degree of endurance in the Tarahumara was leg pain rather than any lung or heart symptoms. Dr. Dale Groom, who has examined and observed these people, summarized in the *American Heart Journal*

(March 1971) that "the phenomenal feats of physical endurance of these primitive Indian runners afford convincing evidence that most of us, brought up in our sedentary, comfortable civilization of today, actually develop and use only a fraction of our potential cardiac reserve."

10

Smoke gets in your heart

Unquestionably, the human being has a phenomenal capacity for exercise. Unfortunately, too many of us abuse our bodies and markedly reduce this tremendous capacity, developing clinical symptoms like fatigue and shortness of breath. Another prevalent abuse in our society is the inhalation of smoke, either as a result of air pollution or through such habits as cigarette, pipe, or cigar smoking, or marijuana usage.

Cigarettes, cigars, pipes

There have been extensive studies showing a definite correlation between smoking and heart disease. A dose-response curve has been established from the National Cooperative Pooling Project, indicating that the man who smokes over one pack per day has twice the risk of developing a coronary event than the one-half-pack per day smoker. Those who quit smoking in the past had only a slight increase in heart attack incidence as compared to the non-smoker, raising the possibility of a causal association and giving encouragement to those in the medical profession who actively speak out against the smoking habit. The highest death rates from coronary disease in the smokers occurred in the younger age group, making this group a target for a preventive cardiology education.

The mechanism by which cigarette smoking aggravates or accelerates the process of atherosclerosis appears to be at least twofold. Nicotine stimulates the release of catecholamines (such as epinephrine) from the adrenal gland, resulting in the elevation of heart rate and blood pressure, and thereby increasing the oxygen requirements of heart muscle. Cardiac rhythm disorders may also be induced. Patients with angina pectoris had a significant decrease in their exercise tolerance after smoking just one cigarette (either high or low in nicotine content). As a result, Dr. Wilbert Aronow and coworkers in Long Beach, California, studied the effects of nonnicotine, lettuce-leaf cigarettes to see whether they too impaired exercise performance.

Ten men with angina pectoris each smoked eight lettuce-leaf cigarettes over a duration of several hours and then exercised on a bicycle ergometer. Unlike nicotine cigarettes, the lettuce variety did not significantly affect the resting blood pressure or heart rate. It did, however, cause a significant elevation in the blood carboxyhemoglobin level (the amount of carbon monoxide which attaches to the red blood cells). Since carbon monoxide has a much greater affinity for hemoglobin than does oxygen, it tends to displace the latter and interfere with oxygen delivery to the tissues. As a result, patients with angina pectoris developed chest pain sooner after exercise since the oxygen demands of heart muscle could not be met. Nonsmokers have blood carboxyhemoglobin levels of 0.4 percent as opposed to the range of 3–10 percent in cigarette smokers. While the effect of this may not be apparent to the person with a normal heart, it can be a definite hindrance to the patient with coronary disease. Since exposure to carbon monoxide accelerates the rate of atherosclerosis in the experimental animal, it is of further concern to man.

It appears, then, that at least two ingredients of cigarettes are harmful. Nicotine increases the oxygen needs of heart muscle, while carbon monoxide interferes with oxygen delivery to the muscle. Together, they form a potentially lethal combination, particularly in the individual whose coronary disease already impairs blood (and hence oxygen) delivery to heart muscle. There are many areas that need further investigation. For instance, smokers have a greater risk of sudden death than nonsmokers, but the reasons for this are not immediately apparent. One possible explanation is a nicotine-induced fatal heart rhythm disturbance. In view of the recent advertising campaign advocating cigar and pipe smoking, we need to know more about these effects on the cardiovascular system. The risk of developing a fatal heart attack is less for pipe or cigar smokers than for cigarette smokers; however, one study reported a significant increased risk for nonfatal heart attacks in cigar and pipe smokers. Coronary risks for ex-smokers approached the nonsmoker rates, as evidenced by epidemiology studies in Framingham, Massachusetts, Albany, New York, and in England. Among the British physicians who gave up cigarettes, the death rates from coronary disease decreased by 7 percent, whereas there was a 35 percent increase in the same rate for the general population. The duration of time necessary to reduce the coronary risk appreciably after cessation of smoking also needs further investigation. While some feel that it takes less than a year to decrease the risk, others provide data suggesting that it may take ten years or more for heavy, chronic smokers.

Marijuana

Marijuana has the effect of increasing heart rate. This has been variously ascribed to an excitation of the central nervous system, to sympathetic nervous system stimulation, or to parasympathetic inhibition. Peter Beaconsfield and his associates at the Royal Free Hospital Medical School, London, recently studied the effects of marijuana on ten healthy volunteer doctors. Similar to tobacco, marijuana increased the heart rate in the subjects, but unlike tobacco, it did not increase levels of blood sugar, lactic acid, and certain fatty acids. Furthermore, marijuana augmented the flow of blood to the arms and muscles and interfered with certain blood vessel reflexes. As a result, in an emergency the fight-or-flight reflex blood vessel response might be impaired. Also, the use of local anesthetics (containing epinephrine) or presurgical medication with an antiparasympathetic drug (like atropine) might seriously augment the underlying rapid heart rate in a marijuana smoker. Marijuana can also affect the electrocardiogram, causing changes which could be mistaken for ischemia of heart muscle. The levels of systolic and diastolic blood pressure were elevated by ten and five mm Hg respectively in the volunteer physicians, and this effect lasted for one-half hour. While this elevation would not be significant in a person with normal blood pressure, it could be undesirable in an already hypertensive person.

Wilbert Aronow and John Cassidy, physicians at Long Beach Veterans Administration Hospital, studied the effects of ten puffs of smoke from the marijuana cigarette on ten men with coronary heart disease and found that exercise tolerance was significantly decreased as a result, probably due to impaired oxygen delivery and/or increased oxygen requirements of heart muscle.

Air pollution

Air pollution has not been given serious study in terms of its effect upon heart function until relatively recently. One of the most interesting studies was done by a group of California investigators—Dr. Wilbert Aronow and associates performed baseline blood studies, electrocardiograms, and exercise tests on ten patients with angina pectoris. The patients were then driven through heavy Los Angeles freeway traffic for ninety minutes in a station wagon with all the windows rolled down. The electrocardiogram was monitored continuously during the driving period. All of the baseline studies were duplicated immediately after the freeway driving. Three weeks later the patients underwent the same procedures with one major exception: they breathed purified compressed air from a tank through a mask. The results were striking. Three of the ten patients developed changes on the electrocardiograms while breathing freeway air that were indicative of inadequate blood supply to the heart muscle. No such changes developed when breathing the purified air. Exercise performance, lung function studies, and the blood-pressure heart-rate product (a measure of energy requirement of the heart muscle) also decreased after breathing the freeway air. Some of these changes involve the amount of carbon monoxide in the blood stream. It was increased from a mean of 1.12 percent to a mean value of 5.08 percent after breathing freeway air. After breathing the purified air, the arterial levels of carboxyhemoglobin actually fell from a baseline of 0.83 percent to 0.65 percent. We have previously seen that carbon monoxide causes the red blood cells to be stingy with oxygen release, an act which is detrimental to the heart muscle that relies so strongly on oxygen for its energy production.

It has been estimated that 20 billion pounds of carbon monoxide were emitted by Los Angeles motor vehicles per day during 1967. Certainly more investigation is needed, and soon, to substantiate and further the work of Aronow and associates, for the air we breathe may be just as deadly as the cigarette smoke we inhale.

11

Hypertension: The silent killer

"But doctor," said Phil Chambers, a forty-six-year-old executive, "how can I have high blood pressure when I feel so well?" This question has been asked in physicians' offices everywhere. In spite of the educational efforts of the American Heart Association, the majority of people still don't understand that hypertension is indeed a silent killer. One can feel perfectly well and have blood pressure readings as high as 240/140 mm Hg. The deleterious effects of high pressure on the so-called target organs, such as the brain, heart, eyes, and kidneys, often occur in the absence of symptoms. These develop when the target organ has been severely compromised. Indeed, the first clue to underlying hypertension might be the sudden onset of a cerebrovascular accident (i.e., stroke) or perhaps a heart attack.

Definition

What is hypertension? Blood pressure screening teams—consisting of medical personnel working in conjunction with the local Heart Association—often give questionnaires to those being screened and frequently get a vast array of answers. It is surprising how many people fail to realize that hypertension means high blood pressure. Many say that hypertension is a condition wherein one is under a lot of stress and nervous tension.

To the physiologist, the systolic blood pressure reflects the pressure head that is transmitted throughout the arterial system when the heart contracts, squeezing blood out of its ventricular chambers. The diastolic blood pressure is that pressure within the arteries when the heart is filling with blood from its venous reservoir. The normal systolic blood pressure is less than 140 mm Hg, as measured with a blood pressure cuff or sphygmomanometer. The normal diastolic blood pressure is less than 90 mm Hg. The blood pressure is generally written with the systolic blood pressure on the top and the diastolic blood pressure on the bottom (as 140/90 mm Hg). As people age the arteries lose some of their elasticity and this has the effect of increasing the resistance and the blood pressure, particularly the systolic reading. Hence, it is not unusual for a seventy-year-old person to have a systolic blood pressure of 160 mm Hg. While this reading is considered elevated by most standards, it is of much less concern than a similar reading in a twenty-five-year-old.

Cause

What causes hypertension? The person who correctly answers that question will be first in line for a Nobel Prize. In over 85–90 percent of cases of hypertension, the cause (or etiology) is unknown. Many use the term *essential hypertension* to describe it. This is merely a term to indicate that there is no evidence for the known causes of hypertension.

What are some of the known causes? Several different tumors in the adrenal gland, which rests like a crown atop the kidneys, can produce hormones in excess, with one of the end results being the development of hypertension. The kidneys can be the source, as well as the target, of hypertension, through the production of substances named renin and prostaglandin. Overproduction or lack of production of such substances due to occlusions of a renal artery, renal damage from repeated infections, and the like can result in the onset of hypertension. Research into the cause (more likely *causes*) of hypertension has been intensified over the past few years and it is hopeful that answers will be forthcoming.

One must realize that blood pressure fluctuates tremendously over a twenty-four-hour period. This must be kept in mind by physicians and patients alike before embarking on a lengthy (and often expensive) course of investigation and therapy. The pressure declines during evening hours and rises either acutely or gradually during the early hours of the day. The systolic pressure in normal people will vary up to 33 mm Hg during the course of a day, while the diastolic pressure varies up to 10 mm Hg or more. Emotional factors also affect blood pressure. The mere presence of a physician may elevate the pressure by 15 mm Hg or more. While the blood pressure in most people tends to increase with age, this is not the case in people everywhere.

Prevalence

Hypertension has become the most prevalent cardiovascular disease in the United States. A survey in Framingham, Massachusetts, initiated twenty years ago on over 5000 men and women, indicated that 18 percent of the men and 16 percent of the women had blood pressure elevations greater than 160/95 mm Hg. Also of significance was the discovery that 41 percent of the men and 48 percent of the women had levels in excess of 140/90 mm Hg. Insurance companies have long been aware that blood pressure levels serve as a predictor of longevity.

In 1962 the National Health Survey estimated that approximately 26 million Americans were hypertensive and the majority were probably not even aware of the problem. Efficient community blood pressure screening teams will help, but such programs are inadequate without proper follow-up.

An illustration of the current sad state of hypertension detection, therapy, and follow-up can be seen in the community screening project which was recently completed in Baldwin County, Georgia. Drs. Joseph Wilber and Gordon Barrow, who headed the investigations, reported that for every one hundred persons screened, twenty-five were found to be hypertensive. Of the twenty-five only sixteen will even reach a physician for diagnosis and treatment. Of the sixteen who do so, only half will adhere to the treatment programs and only one-fourth will achieve adequate blood pressure control for a one-year period. To put it another way, only four of every twenty-five hypertensive persons (16 percent) are being adequately treated. These data, of course, come from a single study in one county, but experience in other centers makes it likely that these statistics have much wider application.

For example, the hypertension screening survey in Chicago revealed similar data. Of 4625 persons found to be hypertensive, only 11.2 percent had a reduction to normal levels after having drug therapy. It is not fair to blame this failure on the drugs utilized, because at present there is a vast array of available drugs—ranging from the mild to the potent. The mild drugs include tranquilizers (such as phenobarbital) and diuretics (which facilitate water removal from the body). The stronger agents block some of the effects of the nervous system on the arteries. It would appear that patients need to be more reliable in taking their medication and in keeping regular appointments. Likewise, physicians need to be more diligent in supervising their patients' compliance to a given therapy regimen.

One of the obstacles that physicians face in treating high blood pressure is the fact that many patients think they can tell when their pressure is increased; hence, they may ignore the prescription instructions and take the drugs only when they feel that their pressure is high. Nervousness, nosebleeds, headaches, and ear-ringing are some of the symptoms these patients use to determine their need for medical treatment.

In a health examination survey headed by Dr. Noel Weiss of the National Center for Health Statistics in Rockville, Maryland, close questioning of 6672 subjects showed absolutely no relationship between blood pressure levels and the presence of nosebleeds, ear-ringing, or headaches. Only in patients with very high levels of diastolic blood pressure was a correlation made with the symptoms of dizziness.

Importance of control

Why is it important to control high blood pressure? For one thing, a fourteen-year follow-up analysis of the Framingham data revealed that the risk of stroke from cerebrovascular thrombosis is directly related to the blood pressure level. Blood pressure control is particularly important in women. Prior to the age of menopause, women have half the incidence of coronary disease of men. However, those with hypertension have the same risk as men! While it was formerly thought that only diastolic hypertension was of importance, the Framingham study has made it clear that systolic hypertension by itself is a risk factor for coronary heart disease. In fact, for all the women in the study, and for men older than forty-five, it was a stronger determinant of future coronary events than was the diastolic blood pressure.

Another reason for strict control of hypertension pertains to heart failure. In a sixteen-year follow-up of a population sample numbering 5192 persons, the onset of heart failure was preceded by hypertension in 75 percent of the cases. The heart failure, which appeared as a consequence of long-standing high blood pressure, markedly shortened the life span. Half of the patients in this category died within five years after the first signs of heart failure appeared. Clearly, early detection and a vigorous follow-up therapy program of change in diet plus drugs could have saved (or at least prolonged) many of those lives.

Other organs which are ravaged by poorly controlled hypertension include the eyes and kidneys. The retinal arteries become thickened, tortuous, and narrowed in long-standing moderate hypertension. In severe hypertension one may see hemorrhages in the retina and swelling of the optic nerve disc, resulting in visual impairment. The small arteries in the kidneys can undergo concentric thickening (so-called onion-skin thickening). Such changes can eventually lead to hemorrhages and scar tissue formation within the kidneys, the ultimate result being renal failure.

Ordinarily the large arteries that carry blood from the right side of the heart to the lungs (the pulmonary arteries) are not involved in atherosclerosis. If the pressure within this artery is increased (so-called pulmonary hypertension, the cause of which is often due to congenital heart disease or lung problems), the same type of "hardening" or atherosclerosis will develop. This finding lends support to those who contend that elevated levels of blood pressure within the coronary arteries and aorta predispose these same vessels to premature, accelerated atherosclerosis.

What evidence exists that control of elevated blood pressure will decrease the risks of stroke, heart failure, and coronary disease? The Veterans Admin-

istration conducted well-controlled studies on 380
men whose diastolic blood pressure ranged from 90
to 114 mm Hg. The patients were randomly assigned
to either an active drug treatment group or to a
placebo group (treated with inert tablets). Over a
five-year follow-up period, there were nineteen
deaths in the placebo group versus eight deaths in
the drug treatment group. Morbid events (stroke,
heart attack, heart failure, etc.) developed in 55 percent of the placebo group and in only 18 percent of
the treated group. The drug treatment seemed more
effective in preventing strokes and heart failure than
for preventing the various complications of coronary
heart disease.

Summary

Getting back to Phil Chambers, the
forty-six-year-old executive with hypertension, he
has a common disease. It frequently exists without
visible symptoms. The cause is largely unknown.
Effective drugs are available to treat the disease, but
such treatment is often thwarted by patient unre-
liability and physician apathy. Damage to target
organs such as the brain, heart, kidney, and eye is
commonplace. There is evidence that such damage
can be appreciably decreased by adequate blood pressure control. The ingredients of the latter are a faith-
ful patient, an interested physician, and effective
medications.

Unfortunately, Phil Chambers did not heed the
advice of his physician. Despite intensive educational
efforts by his physician and his nurse, Phil was too
caught up in the "hurry-sickness" of being a corpo-

rate executive to pay proper attention to his disease. He missed appointments, often let his medication run out without asking for a refill, and took the medication haphazardly. At age fifty, he experienced the first of a series of strokes that were to render him totally disabled, the victim of a disease that can and should be held in check.

The cholesterol hypothesis

Cholesterol has recently become a household word. Literally thousands of medical and lay articles have expounded on the possible relationship between this four-membered benzene ring structure and the development of coronary artery disease. Countless dollars have been spent to finance laboratory investigations as to whether or not dietary intake of cholesterol and other saturated or animal fats (found in such foods as eggs, whole milk, butter, cheese, and beef) and blood levels of cholesterol are related to premature coronary artery disease.

In spite of the above efforts, the public and many members of the medical community themselves remain confused about the whole issue. What is the cholesterol hypothesis? What recent insights and breakthroughs have been made?

Richard Podell, M.D., has nicely summarized the hypothesis in the January 1974 issue of the *American Family Practice Journal*:

1. Blood cholesterol levels can be used to predict the risk of future coronary disease.
2. Blood cholesterol levels can be reduced by decreasing the amount of cholesterol and saturated fat in the diet.
3. Blood cholesterol is directly and causally related to the development of coronary heart disease.
4. By lowering the levels of blood cholesterol through diet and/or drugs, the subsequent risk of coronary disease can be reduced.

The first component of the cholesterol hypothesis has been supported by the American Heart Association in its *Coronary Risk Handbook*, available to physicians. The handbook is based on the research data from the Framingham Study. Based on a person's age, sex, smoking habits, systolic blood pressure level, blood sugar, cholesterol level, and resting electrocardiogram (ECG), one can get an index of coronary risk over the next six-year period. For example, a fifty-year-old male cigarette smoker with a normal blood sugar and resting ECG and systolic blood pressure of 150 mm Hg has a 6.6 percent risk of developing a coronary within six years, if his serum cholesterol level is 185 mg percent. On the other hand, if his blood cholesterol level is 335 mg percent, his risk is nearly three times as great.

While the Framingham data supplied positive answers to the first part of the hypothesis, they did not contribute to the second part about dietary habits. However, other epidemiological studies, such as the New York Anti-Coronary Club dietary approach, have shown that by limiting cholesterol and saturated fat intake, the serum cholesterol level can be reduced. In most similar studies, this reduction has been around 15 percent.

Experimental data on animals suggest that the third component of the hypothesis is correct; namely that cholesterol in the blood is a direct cause of coronary heart disease. By increasing the amount of cholesterol in the diet of rhesus monkeys, investigators have been able to induce coronary disease. If the diet is then changed to a low-cholesterol variety, the coronary lesions regress. Adequate data on humans to corroborate this are lacking, although investigators at the University of California in Davis have documented appreciable improvement in leg blood flow following three to six months of blood lipid-lowering treatment. In other words, the fatty deposits in the leg arteries apparently lessened, thereby increasing blood flow through the vessels.

The fourth component of the hypothesis was alluded to in Chapter 2. Data from the New York Anti-Coronary Club members, Los Angeles veterans, Finnish mental hospital patients, and the Chicago Coronary Prevention Evaluation program all indicated a reduced risk of coronary disease when appropriate dietary modifications were made. These early studies are not without flaws, however, and it is hoped that second generation studies of a similar nature can correct these minor defects in study design so that more meaningful data can be accumulated.

Triglycerides and lipoprotein types

While considerable attention has been given to the role of cholesterol in the development of atherosclerosis, it has only been recently that another type of blood fat, namely the triglycerides, has come under scrutiny. Animal fats contain triglyceride, and carbohydrates are converted in the body into triglycerides, which are complex molecules comprised of glycerol, fatty acids, and monoglycerides. The triglycerides are broken down into these component parts within the intestinal tract. The monoglycerides are taken up by the intestinal cell wall, and triglyceride is again formed. The latter then links up with phospholipid and protein, becoming a complex molecular structure called a chylomicron. The chylomicron is transported through lymphatic channels to the liver or can be taken up by the adipose (fat) tissue of the body. Almost 90 percent of adipose tissue is comprised of triglyceride, which represents a reservoir of stored energy for the body. Since the formation of triglyceride is facilitated by glucose, a high carbohydrate diet may result in a high blood triglyceride level.

About 50 percent of the lipid (or fat) in blocked areas of the coronary arteries consists of triglyceride. Since a number of relatively young persons with elevated blood triglyceride levels experience early signs and symptoms of coronary disease, many epidemiologists have become interested in studying the possible cause and effect relationship between triglycerides and coronary disease in various population groups.

Donald Fredrickson, M.D., and coworkers at the National Heart and Lung Institute have identified five different types of blood fat abnormalities.

In the Type I disorder, both the blood cholesterol and the triglyceride levels are high, the latter sometimes reaching levels over 1000 mg percent, which is seven times higher than normal. Similar elevations can be seen in the Type V disorder. The Type II pattern involves either excessive cholesterol production in the body or inadequate breakdown of cholesterol. Mild abnormalities of this type are often related to improper diet, whereas more severe problems often indicate a genetic (or hereditary) predisposition. In view of the latter, it is of utmost importance to look for this abnormality in all close relatives of an afflicted individual. The Type III pattern can sometimes be spotted by the fatty deposits which form in the palms of the hands. The final pattern, Type IV, can often be missed if the physician does not routinely order a blood triglyceride level test, for the latter will be high while the cholesterol will be normal. This type responds to decreases in carbohydrate consumption and to weight reduction. It may also be modified by exercise.

For cases that do not respond to the simple measures of diet, weight reduction, and exercise, drug therapy may be prescribed. For example, the drug of choice for a Type II pattern is Questran, which combines with intestinal blood fats and impairs their absorption. Type IV disorders, on the other hand, respond better to Atromid-S, an agent that seems to interfere with production of the lipids within the body. Atromid-S may have additional beneficial effects, such as the reduction of blood platelet stickiness. This might decrease blood clot formation within the coronary arteries.

Coronary occlusion

If cholesterol and triglycerides are significant contributors to coronary atherosclerosis, by what means do they get into the walls of the coronary arteries? The lipid infiltration theory, postulated by outstanding pathologists, suggests an active process by which the lipoproteins are transported across the inner lining cells of the arteries. In support of this theory is the recent finding that radioactive-labeled cholesterol, injected into preterminal patients (with their consent), has been recovered within the lining of the aorta. Cholesterol and triglycerides are found in fatty streaks and fibrous plaques, both of which are precursors of the atherosclerotic plaque. Interestingly, concentrations of cholesterol within the plaque are similar to cholesterol concentrations within the blood stream.

Another mechanism under consideration is the thrombogenic theory, which presupposes that small blood clots occur on the surface of the arterial lining cells, attracting red blood cells, platelets, and blood fats. These substances are subsequently incorporated into the wall of the blood vessel. This theory does not explain the mechanism of the latter deposition, nor does it explain the occasional presence of severe atherosclerosis in persons with blood-clotting deficiencies. Still another consideration is the vascular dynamics theory, which suggests that the angulation and curvature of the coronary arteries and their branches produces a mechanical irritation on the vessel walls, setting in motion the process of fibrous thickening and lipid deposition. A fourth theory is the capillary hemorrhage theory which supposes that the tiny blood vessels which nourish the walls of the arteries may rupture, releasing blood fats and other material that can deposit inside the wall of the larger artery.

Current approach

In the face of controversy, pure theory, and physician debate, what guidelines should a person follow? One can summarize all this by saying that blood cholesterol levels can be reduced by diet and drug therapy. Although proof is still lacking that high levels of blood cholesterol per se cause coronary atherosclerosis, the evidence from available studies suggests that the risk of this disease can be reduced by lowering the blood levels of cholesterol. Although data implicating triglycerides as a coronary risk factor are still somewhat scanty, the fact that triglycerides are present in coronary plaques and the finding of premature coronary disease in certain young persons with significant elevations of serum triglycerides make it prudent to lower the blood triglyceride levels when elevated.

Some contend that drastic measures of dietary and blood fat manipulations are not indicated in the absence of clear-cut evidence of cause and effect. But is it really drastic to reduce egg consumption to three per week, to substitute skim milk for whole milk, or to eat more fish and poultry instead of steak and roasts? Is it really drastic to exercise in moderation (as little as ninety minutes per week) and to maintain optimal body weight? It would hardly seem so, particularly in a country that faces an epidemic of coronary disease, an epidemic that could probably be curtailed.

13

How personality
and behavior
affect the heart

The wise physician does not treat disease or organ systems, but rather treats the whole man. In so doing, the impact of a disease, especially cardiac, on the psyche is of utmost importance in determining the best form of overall therapy. The impact of an emotional disorder on a particular organ system becomes important when one attempts to separate the symptoms which are related to nervousness from those which reflect a serious organic disease such as cancer or heart disease.

Sudden death and psychological stress

Dr. Roy J. Shephard of the University of Toronto's School of Hygiene has shown that "the intensity of stress imposed upon the heart by an

119

anxiety reaction may exceed that incurred during maximum exercise." In 1971, the *Annals of Internal Medicine* published (with some reservations) a provocative article entitled "Sudden and Rapid Death During Psychological Stress." Since sudden death is almost always cardiovascular in origin, the relationship between emotional strain and the heart becomes a very serious consideration. In this article, George Engel of the Department of Psychiatry and Medicine of the University of Rochester School of Medicine has gathered 170 examples of death directly related to one of the following eight acute stress settings:

1. Collapse or death of a close person
2. A period of acute grief
3. Threat of loss of a close person
4. Mourning or anniversary of the death of a close person
5. A sudden loss of status or self-esteem
6. Personal danger or the threat of injury, real or symbolic
7. The period following such danger
8. A reunion, triumph, or happy ending

Ninety-nine instances involved men, most of whom were between forty-five and fifty-five. Women were generally older, with the peak period being seventy to seventy-five. Parallels were drawn with animals whose deaths were observed during a period of intense fear, transfer to an unfamiliar environment, or following the loss of a mate. The autonomic nervous system, which can induce heart rhythm disturbances, is believed to be the most likely underlying mechanism of death.

Psychological factors

Lawrence Perlman of the Medical College of Wisconsin and his associates have pointed out the importance of social and emotional factors in precipitating heart failure. In a series of 105 cases, acute emotional events preceded hospitalization in fifty-one cases. These events included threats to independence, separation, anxious anticipation, change in usual routine, and emotional outbursts.

Henry Russek, a New York cardiologist, was able to correlate a job-related emotional upheaval with the onset of coronary heart disease in 91 out of 100 patients—most of whom were relatively young. Others have written about psychological hazards that appear after the onset of coronary disease. Psychiatric difficulties occur in anywhere from 30 to 70 percent of those who are confined in intensive care units. Six out of sixty patients admitted to a coronary care unit were delirious at some time. Forty of the sixty cases were extremely anxious, while twenty-nine admitted to bouts of depression. During long-term convalescence from a myocardial infarction, emotional problems can seriously interfere with the rehabilitation process and the return to work. In a group of twenty-four patients treated at the Massachusetts General Hospital, twenty-one were either anxious or depressed and eighteen required medication. Sixteen patients reported family quarrels directly attributed to some aspect of their convalescence. Fifteen patients complained of sleep disturbances. Of eleven patients who did not return to work, nine failed to return for psychological reasons.

Considerable research has attempted to relate

social variables to coronary heart disease. In an exhaustive review of 154 papers, it was found that the relationship between incidence of and death rates from coronary disease and such factors as population density, national level of education, religion, income, marital status, and occupation was not yet very clear. Other research has come up with more interesting, albeit somewhat incongruous, results. An autopsy study in Israel showed correlation of the extent of atherosclerosis to the variables of occupation, education, and size of the home. It was found that those who had larger homes and more education also had more atherosclerosis. In Chile, there was likewise a higher degree of coronary disease in men of upper socioeconomic status and in those doing primarily intellectual work.

Two studies from the New York area provided interesting contrasts. In the Health Insurance Plan members, white-collar workers had more coronary disease than the blue-collar workers. However, when the two groups were matched up regarding their physical activity levels, no significant differences in coronary disease rates were present. In the New York Bell Telephone System, the level of education seemed inversely related, in that death rates from coronary disease were twice as high in high school graduates as in college men. The Western Electric study also reported higher rates of myocardial infarction and sudden death in men with less education. Strangely enough, chest pain due to coronary disease (angina pectoris) was more prevalent in the better educated, somewhat clouding the issue.

In the early 1960s a medical team from the University of Oklahoma became interested in the Italian-

American community of Roseto, Pennsylvania. This community had only half the coronary death rate of Bangor, a small city of mixed ethnic groups located only one mile away. The Roseto inhabitants consumed higher than average amounts of calories and of saturated fats, had poor exercise habits, and were generally overweight. The Oklahoma team suggested that perhaps it was their happy-go-lucky, low-key lifestyle that protected them against coronary disease.

Social mobility and uncomfortable job demands have been evaluated in several studies as possible contributing factors toward premature coronary heart disease. In a comparative study from Nazareth, Pennsylvania, individuals with coronary heart disease had frequently moved from place to place. Furthermore, they were more often involved in a job that demanded an educational level higher than they possessed, thereby leading to feelings of inferiority and insecurity. In the Trappist-Benedictine monk evaluation, migration from a low socioeconomic background to a higher level seemed to constitute a risk factor. There were more heart attacks in those monks with a college education who came from families of low socioeconomic level. In the Western Electric Study, which involved 1472 men, several aspects of social status were assessed—income, religion, level of education, occupation, size of home, type of neighborhood, and membership in voluntary organizations.

As a general rule, the higher status was again associated with a higher risk of developing coronary disease. Elevated risk was also apparent in men whose educational level was not equal to that of their spouse.

Several types of questionnaires are available for use in quantifying levels of anxiety and neuroticism. One such test, the Minnesota Multiphasic Personality Inventory, is used routinely in schools, hospitals, and clinics. A. M. Ostfeld found that persons who scored high on neurotic scales of hypochondriasis, depression, and hysteria tended to develop coronary heart disease at an accelerated rate. Ancel Keys and Henry Blackburn, researchers at the University of Minnesota, confirmed this and added a strong masculine behavior pattern as an indication of higher risk. Low levels of hostility, as compared to higher tendencies toward anxiety and regression, appeared of importance in assessing future coronary risk according to M. A. Ibrahim, but this could not be confirmed by other investigators. Despite the incongruities between the various studies, most had at least one consistency—before the onset of illness, patients with coronary heart disease scored higher on the neurotic triad (hysteria, depression, and hypochondriasis) than did those without this disease. Curiously, persons who developed angina pectoris alone had worse scores on the triad than did those who developed myocardial infarctions.

The 16 Personality Factor Inventory is shorter than the MMPI (144 questions as opposed to 544) but yields equally interesting data. In the Western Electric Study, those who were later to develop coronary disease tended to be more suspicious and jealous, had greater feelings of inner tension, and were more self-sufficient and independent than those free of disease. Similarly, patients with angina pectoris tended to be more emotionally unstable than those with myocardial infarctions. In a retrospective study involving 112 men, C. P. Bakker and R. M. Levenson found the coronary patients to be conformists, somber, prudish, and compulsive. Once again, the patients with angina pectoris alone were less stable, more conforming, less conscientious, more timid and apprehensive, and more hung-up on inner urgencies than the infarction patients. Why these two groups should differ psychologically remains an enigma since the underlying coronary disease process (i.e., atherosclerosis) remains the same. A tendency to be compulsive and precise was noted in studies of the Trappist-Benedictine monks who developed coronary heart disease. However, the same group also tended to be both outgoing and easy going, warm-hearted, venturesome, and uninhibited, qualities that one would not ordinarily attribute to coronary proneness. In general, the two tests seem to corroborate that the coronary candidate is often beset beforehand by emotional troubles.

Personality types

A possible breakthrough in our understanding of the brain-heart interaction occurred in 1959, the year that Drs. Ray Rosenman and Meyer Friedman described two specific personality types in their articles in medical journal reports. Type A were tense, highly competitive persons who drove themselves hard to achieve self-designated (and usually poorly defined) goals. This type of person actually enjoys job-related deadlines as he strives for personal recognition and job advancement. He or she has a tendency to accelerate both mental and physical functions, with bursts of rapid speech and a desire to perform each task quickly. This person goes all-out even in a friendly card or ping-pong game. He or she will be irritated by a slow driver, and, though quick to anger, will usually conceal the emotion. He or she generally will attempt to accomplish other work while eating or while on the toilet. If a speaker takes too long to get to the point, he will be inclined to interrupt in an effort to hurry him along. A man might even go to such extremes as buying several electric shavers in an endless quest to shave faster. This type, when asked to hold the line after dialing a phone number, will usually hang up in several seconds and dial again.

Type B, on the other hand, has nearly opposite traits. He or she is unlikely to become irritated when waiting in a movie or restaurant line. He or she may have participated in school activities, but did not strive to lead. These people don't worry about being on time, and, in fact, probably wouldn't hurry especially to catch the kickoff of a football game. These researchers also used a third group as a control, consisting of forty-six blind men who were in a chronic state of anxiety and insecurity. Strangely enough, one's chances of being classical Type A are no greater for a bank president than a janitor.

In the Western Collaborative Group Study, 3295 men were classified as having either Type A or Type B behavior patterns, based on the results of an interview and a questionnaire. The Type A individual is not hard to spot in the interview, for he often has a rapid, forceful speech pattern and frequently punctuates his points with a clenched fist, by pointing his finger, or by pounding on a desk top. The study classified 1664 men as Type A and 1631 as Type B.

In a follow-up study, Type A persons developed coronary disease at a rate six times greater than Type B. In the fifty-one cases who died and were evaluated on the autopsy table, the extent of coronary atherosclerosis was six times as severe in Type A. No significant group differences existed regarding cigarette consumption, dietary pattern, exercise habits, or blood pressure levels. By using a special mathematical formula (the multiple regression equation), it was shown that when twelve risk factors were statistically controlled, the relationship of behavior pattern to the frequency and extent of coronary disease still existed in the younger patients. In similar studies involving 1500 Trappist and Benedictine monks, the rate of heart attack was four times greater in Type A than in B. Several Boston investigators administered the Rosenman-Friedman test to a group of patients who were hospitalized with coronary heart disease and with other chronic disorders. He found more Type A personalities among the coronary group than in the noncoronary group.

The findings of Rosenman and Friedman take on added significance with the discovery that the Type A individual also had these associated abnormalities:

1. Higher serum cholesterol levels
2. More rapid blood clotting times
3. Higher levels of urinary adrenalin excretion
4. Higher serum triglyceride levels (before and after fatty food intake)

5. Higher blood insulin responses to an oral sugar intake
6. Lower growth hormone levels
7. *Sludging* of blood in the tiny conjunctival eye vessels (which may persist for up to nine hours after a high-fat meal)

By using the above information, one can come up with a scheme which ties together the psychosocial factors with the biochemical and pathological factors:

Both hereditary and environmental factors result in a specific personality and behavior pattern. The Type A person possesses the tendency to higher blood fat levels, labile high blood pressure, excessive sympathetic nervous system discharge, faster blood clotting, and sludging of blood in small vessels, factors which combine to accelerate the process of coronary atherosclerosis until clinical symptoms of angina pectoris or a myocardial infarction appear.

This is, no doubt, an oversimplification of the complex process of atherosclerosis and additional studies from other centers are needed to corroborate the initial observations of Rosenman and Friedman.

How to modify Type A

What can the extreme Type A person do to modify his or her behavior pattern? There are a dozen relatively simple steps to take, but each requires almost daily practice and repetition before it becomes habit or second nature:

1.   One of the first steps is to refrain from polyphasic thinking, wherein one is continually thinking about two things at one time or has a "flight" of ideas. The best way to accomplish this is to practice total concentration on the events or happenings of a particular moment rather than entertaining thoughts of future problems and possibilities that might never transpire. The anxious person frequently thinks about the various sources of his anxiety to the point where he becomes virtually ineffective at dealing with even one of the aggravating sources.

2.   The Type A person needs time for relaxation, preferably in a scenic outdoor environment. Too many executives pride themselves on the fact that they haven't taken a vacation in years. This is an unhealthy practice and may contribute to premature coronary events. An office briefcase has no place in the vacation suitcase.

3.   Living by a clock must change. It is a cruel irony that the businessman who survives twenty-five years of obsessive clock watching is given—you guessed it—a gold watch upon his retirement. Don't be a clock-watcher. Realize that even if you are five minutes late for an appointment it will make little difference to the 880 million Chinese on the other side of the world.

4.   Talk yourself into relaxing when in certain irritating situations such as waiting for traffic lights. Use self-control and avoid honking the horn, even if it means waiting through another light change.

5.   End the day by reading something enjoyable,

perhaps a good novel or magazine article unrelated to your occupation. Cultivate your interest and appreciation of the arts, be it music, dance, literature, sculpture, or paintings. The Type A person has little time to appreciate the well-written verse, the genius of a Renoir, or the majesty of Beethoven. He or she must take the time!

6. Pay more attention to the world around you. When was the last time that you went out of your way to examine a pretty flower up close or to watch a cardinal busying himself in the backyard?

7. Get plenty of exercise, but enjoy what you do. Don't carry a stopwatch while you jog and don't act like an infant in trying to crush a rival in tennis.

8. Surround yourself with friends that you thoroughly enjoy. Avoid people who irritate you, particularly those who seem adept at bringing out your latent hostility. These people shouldn't be invited to dinner merely because you're indebted to them or because there might be a secondary gain by so doing—it isn't worth it.

9. Savor the taste of fine food instead of challenging the maximum rate that your gastric cells can digest food. Without becoming a bore or a snob, take pride in identifying the grape from whence a tasty wine was derived.

10. Plan your day in advance so you don't have to rush, even if it means getting up thirty minutes earlier in the morning.

11. Be a good listener, particularly to members of your family. The Type A person has little time for some of the seeming trivialities he or she hears in children's conversations, only to wonder later why

the children "never tell me anything" in the difficult teen-age years.

12. Of utmost importance is to know thyself. Periodically review your strengths and your weaknesses and reintensify your efforts to shore up the latter. Live by the Peter Principle by not striving for a job situation that is high in status but low in self-enjoyment. Religious study groups can be of value in the quest for self-assessment and understanding.

At present, the data are insufficient in proving or disproving the theory that behavior modification can reduce cardiac risk. By a better self-understanding, and through professional counseling, it may be possible to control traits and hopefully reduce the risk of premature coronary heart disease. There is little doubt that brain waves interact with heart beats. Man's future survival, along with his sense of well-being, may be greatly influenced by our progress in this fascinating interrelationship.

14

Sexual activity
and the heart

What about sex? Does it have a beneficial effect on cardiac function? Are there any adverse cardiac effects from vigorous sexual activity? When can a postcoronary patient resume sexual intercourse? These are questions frequently asked during cardiac rehabilitation.

Whenever sex is concerned, it is hard to separate fact from fiction. Such is the case when attempting to determine the effects of sexual activity on the cardiovascular system. Recent literature, to use the term loosely, has ranged from the sublime to the ridiculous. The French have described instances of sudden death during sexual intercourse, terming it *la mort d'amour*. One American physician has suggested that frequent sexual activity will produce a cardiac conditioning effect, claiming it to be a pleasurable substitute for exercise regimens. Sex has also been urged as an effective means of losing weight, particularly when substituted for a midnight snack.

A New York cardiologist, Lenore Zohman, indicated that sexual activity is no more stressful for a coronary patient than climbing several flights of stairs, unless it is done outside marital bonds. This prompted the following reply from David Kritchevsky of Philadelphia:

> Coronary, have a care,
> Think, before that new affair.
> Dr. Zohman studied swingers
> And her facts are really zingers.
>
> Sex domestic, also straight,
> Hardly makes you palpitate.
> Heartbeats stay at normal rate
> When one beds with legal mate
> And the dangers that it bears
> Loom like—well, two sets of stairs.
>
> But roosting in another's nest,
> Flirts with cardiac arrest.
> End result of evening's sport is
> Very often rigor mortis.
> So seduction's needs are three—
> Soft lights, music, EKG.

Drs. Hellerstein and Friedman, from Case Western Reserve University, performed a serious study regarding the effect of sexual activity on the electrocardiograms of fourteen postcoronary patients. The electrocardiogram was monitored on an out-patient basis, using an electromagnetic tape recording device. The mean maximal heart rate during peak sexual activity was 117 beats per minute, indeed a level comparable to climbing several flights of stairs. One and two minute postcoital rates were ninety-seven beats per minute and eighty-five beats per minute respectively. Four of the men had chest pain and changes on the electrocardiogram during the activity, indicative of coronary insufficiency, while three had heart rhythm disturbances. Previous reports have indicated that angina-type pain during sexual activity can often be prevented by the prophylactic use of sublingual nitroglycerin. Based upon such data, our postcoronary patients without cardiac symptoms or signs of cardiac rhythm disturbances during in-hospital activities as hall walking and stair climbing are permitted to engage in sexual activity within seven to ten days after returning home. We encourage the patient to play the more passive role in the sexual act for the first two weeks. We initiate the discussion of sexual activity for the hospitalized patients, finding that the latter are often a little embarrased about being the first to bring up the subject. We also encourage questions and comments from the spouse to avoid misunderstandings concerning sex. An example of this is the wife of a rehabilitation patient who refused to have sexual relations with the husband, fearing that it might induce his death. Another example is the wife who resents her husband's impotence after his heart attack, accusing him of not caring about her as much as he once did. Impotence has been relatively infrequent among my patients and usually is quite transitory.

It is difficult to draw conclusions regarding the cardiac stress in sexual activity from relatively small study groups. However, the following are based on available data and common sense:

1. It is unlikely that physical conditioning can be achieved by sexual activity, for the pulse rate, on the average, is not sufficiently elevated and the frequency of activity is less than twice weekly for middle-aged males (according to Kinsey and associates).

2. It is possible for coronary-prone or postcoronary patients to enjoy sexual activity without undue risk. Prophylactic use of nitroglycerin and physical conditioning programs are helpful for those who have cardiac symptoms.

3. It seems highly probable that there will be insufficient cooperation in studying the stress of sex in extramarital affairs.

4. Those who relish variety in life may not wish to substitute sex for vintage wine and quality cuisine in order to shed a few excess pounds.

15

Overweight or overfat?

A serious health problem in the United States is obesity. According to U.S. Public Health statistics, between twenty-five and forty-five percent of our adult population over thirty are more than 20 percent overweight. The prevalence of obesity has greatly increased in the last fifteen years. Sadly enough, approximately 10 million teen-agers, or roughly 20 percent of the total teen-age population, are also overweight.

On the average, an American will add nearly one pound of additional weight each year after twenty-five. While this doesn't seem very dramatic, consider the fifty-five-year-old person who is carrying thirty pounds of excess baggage around with him or her, twenty-four hours a day. Consider also the strain on the heart, which must work so much harder to nourish those unnecessary fat cells.

Insurance companies have emphasized the correlation between overweight and increased mortality from liver and kidney disease, accidents, and cardiovascular disease. Such insurance statistics are based on excess body weight, rather than on excess body fat. This leads the general public to believe that "overweight" is synonymous with "overfat." This is certainly incorrect, for most members of the Atlanta Falcons professional football team are overweight out of necessity for their particular job performance; yet relatively few carry an excess amount of body fat. It has only been in recent years that the complexity of the subject, body weight, has been realized.

To understand aspects of body weight properly, we must separate the two components, excess body weight and excess fat. Most physiologists and nutritionists now feel that it is not how heavy a person becomes that is significant, but how much fat the person carries and how much fat he or she adds per year.

While certain anatomical and chemical methods can be used to determine body composition at autopsy, other methods must be used in the study of living persons. These include such indirect methods for estimating the ratio of lean body mass to body fat such as X-rays of subcutaneous fat, measurement of body density and total body water, and the use of fat-soluble indicators. One of the simplest techniques, and one that carries a high degree of accuracy, is the measurement of skinfold thickness by constant tension skinfold calipers. These represent an advance on the physician's age-old method of simply pinching the patient's skin between thumb and forefinger in an effort to evaluate nutritional status. That technique has suffered from being too haphazard, leading to difficulties in precise measurement and problems in comparative, follow-up measurements.

The use of skinfold calipers has yielded data that correlate well with measurements obtained from X-rays of the body's soft tissues. Such determinations of subcutaneous fat have correlated well with calculations of total body fat obtained by other methods, such as underwater weighing in which lean body mass displaces more water than fat does, based on Archimedes' principle.

Widespread application of the skinfold caliper technique has made it possible to obtain data as to the varying fat content between large numbers of men and women, between persons of different age groups, and between persons who are sedentary and those who are physically active. It has also helped to analyze the overweight person in order to determine whether the overweight is due to an excess in body fat or to an excess in muscle mass. Using the skinfold caliper technique, an adult male should not have more than 14 percent of his total body weight composed of fat. For the adult female, the figure should not exceed 16 percent. Obesity is, by definition, having more than 25 percent of total weight as fat.

Other body components, besides fat and muscle (protein), include water and minerals. While in certain athletes, excess muscle and water contribute appreciably to total body weight, the greatest variable in the body composition of the average American is fat. Indeed, given a group of normal adults of the same height, the individual differences in body weight are largely accounted for by varying amounts of fat tissue.

While skinfold measurement with calipers appears fairly simple, the procedure has been standardized to give it precision. Anywhere from three to ten sites in the body are measured, depending on the method or formula used, but such sites must be meticulously located. One needs to apply firm pressure by the fingers in lifting the skinfold, and the distance that the skinfold is lifted before applying the calipers must be constant, as must the pressure of the calipers itself.

Why not just rely on height and weight charts to determine excess body fat? Researchers in this field have found such charts to be an unreliable predictor of body fatness. The efficiency of predicting body fat from height-weight charts is only 40 percent accurate in young men. In dealing with older patients, the efficiency drops to 23 percent, meaning that one fails to determine body fatness accurately from height-weight charts in four out of five tries.

Causes of obesity

Researchers in animal laboratories have discovered that the region of the brain known as the hypothalamus is the neural regulator of food intake. The portion of the hypothalamus known as the ventromedial nucleus is the satiety center, signaling the body when enough food has been taken in. If this center is purposely destroyed in the animal brain, the result is gross obesity. The lateral region of the hypothalamus is the food-seeking regulator, and surgical damage to this center results in loss of weight and emaciation.

Obesity can be caused by heredity, environment, or a combination of both. Family trends toward obesity have been noted. In one study of 1000 obese children, nearly three-fourths had one or both parents with a similar problem. However, only 9 percent of the children whose parents are average weight will be obese. But which is more important—heredity or environment? If the environmental factor is more important, one would expect adopted children to resemble their foster parents in body composition. This has not been the case in several studies. If heredity plays the major role, identical twins reared in different environments should nonetheless have similar body compositions. Such has been the case, although more studies are needed to provide supportive data.

Social-class standings are found to influence obesity levels in children. Several investigators at the University of Pennsylvania performed skinfold measurements on over 3000 school children in three eastern cities. Obesity was nine times more common by age six in girls of low social class as compared to those of higher class. Similar findings, though to a lesser degree, were noted in boys. Perhaps nutritional misinformation, along with economic deprivation, is responsible for such faulty nutritional status among the lower social classes. Racial factors also merit consideration, for in the southern states one finds more obesity in white men than in white women. The opposite is found in blacks, although some attribute the lesser obesity in black men to their greater physical activity.

A possible breakthrough in our understanding of obesity may come from the laboratory of Dr. Jules Hirsch, a physician at Rockefeller University. Dr. Hirsch estimates that while a lean person has around 27 trillion fat cells in his body, an obese person has three times as many fat cells. Obese persons not only have more fat cells but also have larger individual fat cells, perhaps related to overfeeding in infancy and youth. Dr. Hirsch suggests that such overfeeding can lead to a build up of fat cells that can persist for a lifetime. The large fat cells of an obese person may actually shrink upon weight loss, but the incompletely-filled shrunken cell might in some way initiate a feedback loop to the appetite-center of the brain, creating a powerful stimulus for enhanced food intake which will, in turn, result in an expansion of the cell to its usual size. Hence, overeating may not just be due to psychological factors, but also to physiological factors as well. The fat cell theory has some experimental support in the observation that an animal made obese by damage to the hypothalamic brain area will show an increased size of each individual fat cell (although not an increase in number of cells).

Exercise and overfatness

Dr. Jean Mayer, a Harvard obesity expert, feels that physical inactivity may be a strong contributor to the development of obesity. In observing a multitude of obese persons, Dr. Mayer found that food choices and patterns of eating did not differ significantly, particularly in women. Although often there was a tendency for obese women to consume more of their calories toward the evening hours, the total intake of calories by these women might not exceed that of their lean counterparts. The difference was that the obese persons were much more sedentary than the lean ones and hence used up fewer calories.

Not everyone agrees with Jean Mayer's reasoning. These investigators are quick to point out that since one pound of fat equals 3500 calories, in order to lose this amount of fat one would have to swim for five and one-half hours, cycle for seven and one-half hours, or walk for over eleven hours. They go on to point out the exercise equivalents of several snacks, each consisting of 200 calories. For instance, if you eat two apples you would need to run for twelve consecutive minutes. On the same order, eating eighteen marshmallows would require four hours of dishwashing; the intake of fifty-three peanuts would necessitate singing for three hours to prevent weight gain; and drinking twenty-four ounces of beer would require fourteen hours of television watching.

This way of looking at the relationship between exercise and food intake, while amusing, is not entirely reasonable, for it would certainly discourage an obese person from exercising when the latter would have to be done in ridiculous intensity or duration. However, there is another way of looking at the matter. Since walking for one hour consumes 300 calories, one would expend 2100 calories (or ½ pound of fat) per week walking one hour a day. Over the course of a year, twenty-five pounds of fat would be lost, assuming caloric intake was reasonable. A daily caloric expenditure exceeding the daily intake by 500 calories would result in a weekly fat loss of one pound (or a loss of fifty-two pounds in one year).

Doesn't exercise enhance the appetite? Not necessarily, according to many. Caged animals and relatively immobile people eat more than their active counterparts. Also, rats who were exercised for one to two hours daily ate less food than relatively inactive rats. A time and intensity factor may be involved, for the food intake of rats began to increase if they were exercised for more than two hours daily, provided such exercise did not result in chronic exhaustion, in which case the appetite of the animals fell off and weight was lost.

Age and body fatness

In humans, deposition of body fat occurs predominantly at two ages—early childhood and late maturity. Subcutaneous fat thickness by the skinfold caliper technique increases in infancy, decreases in childhood, and rises again in adulthood. Vertical growth stops in the third decade of life. Too often physical activity also markedly declines in this age group. If appetite and food intake increase, or even if they stay the same, fat storage gradually accrues. The average fat content for men of standard weight differs markedly for various age groups. For instance, at twenty the average fat content is 10.3 percent versus 16.2 percent at thirty, 20.7 percent at forty, and 25 percent at fifty-five. The aging process involves more than just the deposition of fat in the body storage areas; it is also likely that active tissues such as muscle are replaced to some extent by fat and by fibrous tissue.

What to do about obesity

The annals of medical history, particularly the events of the past century, are cluttered with the folly of our attempts at finding an easy way to lose weight. The current rage is the Atkin's Diet, another in the long list of low-carbohydrate diets. Its predecessors included diets by the names of DuPont, Pennington, and Mayo (no kin to the famous clinic). If alcohol is added to such diets, one gets the Drinking Man's Diet, certain to appeal to the masses of American executives and lonely housewives. Other diets have achieved certain popularity, such as the low-protein Rockefeller Diet and the Rice Diet, low in both protein and fat. Over 5 million people purchased copies of the Stillman Diet, consisting almost entirely of protein and animal fat. Few scientific studies accompany such diets and when they do, the side effects of nutritional imbalance can be seen. One example is the study from Harvard on twelve healthy hospital employees who followed the Stillman Diet for an average of one week, losing an average of seven pounds but at the price of increasing their average serum cholesterol level from 215 mg percent to 248 mg percent, a highly significant elevation.

More radical attempts at weight reduction include the surgical procedure known as the small-bowel bypass. By means of the surgery, the small bowel is shortened, causing a smaller surface area of bowel to be available for food absorption. Weight loss by this method, though occasionally dramatic, is often quite variable. Moreover, multiple side effects of the surgery include the risk of operative death, bowel obstruction, water and electrolyte loss, and vitamin deficiency.

The fact remains that there is no easy way to diet and lose weight. The most sensible approach is to eat a balanced diet, consisting of 50 percent carbohydrate, 35 percent fat, and 15 percent protein. The fat should be largely of the polyunsaturated variety. The carbohydrate intake should include limited portions of refined sugar. Obese persons should be urged to eat slowly and to distribute the daily caloric intake over four to six feeding periods to prevent excessive hunger. (One interesting study showed that individuals who ate just one large meal per day had increased cholesterol levels, impaired glucose tolerance, and augmented fat synthesis in adipose tissue.) Since populations accustomed to diets high in fiber have been found to have less colonic disease (including cancer), fewer gallbladder attacks, and a lower incidence of a host of other diseases (ranging from hemorrhoids to hernias), it would seem prudent to increase the amount of fiber in the diet. High in fiber are such foods as bran cereal, raspberries, blueberries, whole wheat breads, raw carrots, and apples.

The above dietary prescription must be accompanied by a sound exercise prescription, one that will provide physical activity, preferably on a daily basis. Patient education is essential to prevent aimless leaping from one fad diet to the next, and follow-up is mandatory. Few diseases require as much motivation and remotivation as does the clinical state of obesity.

16

Alcohol
and the heart

Since a large segment of our population
consumes alcohol in varying amounts, it seems appropriate to review briefly some of the effects of
alcohol on the cardiovascular system.

In the last century, it was felt that alcohol
caused certain instances of heart failure in the absence of nutritional deficiency. In the economic depression period of the 1930s, however, a common
cardiac disorder in alcoholics was beriberi heart disease, caused by a dietary deficiency of vitamin B_1. It
took another twenty to thirty years for physicians to
return to the earlier concept that alcohol itself was
a depressant of heart muscle (myocardial) function.
William Evans, a physician at the London Hospital,
wrote extensively about alcohol-related heart disease. In an article in the *American Heart Journal*

(61:556–67, 1961), he described the typical patient in the following colorful style:

The patient is usually a man past middle age. As a rule, he meets his physician in private rather than in hospital practice. He is neither an outcast of society, a sloth in commerce nor a sluggard in industry, but in fact he is sociable, likeable, loyal and a restless worker. Day in and day out he attends board meetings, directs the destinies of commercial or industrial concerns, canvasses custom and hocks his ware through personal contact when he fills and refills his guest's goblet and his own at the bar or at the table. On his return home he is met with the accumulated work of the day as he opens his briefcase, and he turns to the bottle at his side whose contents he quaffs, either in the hope that they stimulate him to overcome his neglected tasks or in the knowledge that they will help him temporarily to forget them.

Sometimes he is the unhappy husband who has become estranged from his home and prefers to spend his evenings at the club or the bar, thereby avoiding the castigation of his spouse, who sees more clearly than he does the impending doom. He often plays at golf but never excels at it, for he is more engaged in the drinking amenities of the clubhouse than in any attempt to improve his game. He might be an aging bachelor without any hobbies who whiles away his hours of loneliness, and as he attempts to uplift his depressed spirits with alcohol he drains his cup of sorrow in the false hope of removing his own.

The use of alcohol has occasionally been responsible for acute and sometimes fatal heart disease. Several brewers in Canada, Belgium, and the United States began adding cobalt to beer around 1963 in order to make the foam stable. Within several months, multiple episodes of devastating heart disease developed with death rates reaching up to 50 percent. A team of Canadian investigators, using ingenuity that would rival James Bond himself, traced the epidemic to the cobalt additive, thus averting a large-scale epidemic.

The development of cardiac catheterization made it possible to actually quantify various parameters of cardiac function, including the strength of muscle contraction and the amount of blood squeezed out of the heart per beat (stroke volume). The effects of varying amounts of alcohol on the human were then measured.

Dr. Lawrence Gould and colleagues determined the effects of two ounces of Canadian whiskey (the equivalent of several popular cocktails) on the heart. They performed cardiac catheterization studies on ten patients with heart disease and on four normal persons. This amount of alcohol had no appreciable effect in either group on heart rate, blood pressure, and pressure in the blood vessel connecting the right heart chambers to the lungs (i.e., pulmonary artery). All patients with cardiac disease had a reduction in stroke volume, indicative of a detrimental effect on cardiac performance. The normals, on the other hand, actually had a slight increase in this measurement.

Additional studies are forthcoming. At present, the following generalizations can be made:

1. The amount of alcohol in an average cocktail impairs an important aspect of cardiac function, that being the amount of blood pumped per beat, in persons with known heart disease. It has no significant effect on normal individuals.

2. Chronic intake of alcohol, when associated with dietary insufficiencies, leads to the development of a specific type of cardiac malfunction, known as beriberi heart disease.

3. Alcohol abuse (even in the presence of an adequate diet) can lead to cardiac enlargement and failure, disrupting the energy storehouses (mitochondria) within the heart muscle.

4. In the absence of heart disease, prudent use of alcohol does not appear to be detrimental. On the other hand, it may be helpful in that it has a mild tranquilizing effect.

But what constitutes prudent use of alcohol? A number of my preventive cardiology patients have interpreted this to mean two cocktails during the business luncheon and perhaps four or five more around suppertime. This amount is clearly not prudent, for alcohol is high in calories, leading to weight gain, and is also a frequent contributor to high blood triglyceride levels. Moreover, alcohol and exercise make poor companions and the intake of one usually precludes the use of the other. Alcoholism is a growing problem in our country, affecting an estimated 5 to 10 percent of the population. Many got their start by such seemingly innocent alcohol habits as mentioned above.

Wine has been credited with many medical cures, ranging from arthritis to bowel disorders and heart trouble. There are no sound scientific studies to prove any of such outlandish claims. I enjoy learning about various wines, particularly when visiting cardiac rehabilitation centers in such wine meccas as Bordeaux, France, and Freiburg, Germany. When patients inquire about wine, I make it clear to them that it is no panacea for their various medical problems. I advise them to use it in moderation, which does not mean on a daily basis. I also indicate that wine is moderately high in calories, though less so than hard liquor (i.e., three and one-half ounces of Burgundy contains 75 calories, while one and one-half ounces of whiskey has 120 calories).

In summary, much has been learned over the past two decades about the effects of alcohol on the cardiovascular system. There is still a good deal to be discovered about the multiple effects on the various organ systems. At present, it would seem that postcoronary patients should use alcohol sparingly, if at all, limiting themselves to no more than eight drinks per week. The coronary-prone person should likewise be advised to restrict the intake of alcohol and should be channeled into other ways of relaxation and tension-alleviation, such as exercise and self-relaxation breathing exercises.

17

Cardiac rehabilitation

So far, much of this book has emphasized primary prevention or the prevention of the initial episode of coronary disease. It would be remiss not to spend some time in consideration of the person who has already suffered from coronary disease, for nearly one million Americans fall into this category annually. What hope is there for the postcoronary patient? What approach is being used to decrease his or her chances of an untimely death or of a nonfatal recurrent heart attack? Before reflecting upon this let us consider some historical aspects of cardiac rehabilitation.

Historical aspects

One of the earliest notations that exercise might be of benefit in the treatment of coronary patients was made by Dr. William Heberden, who in 1772 stated that one of his patients with coronary insufficiency was "nearly cured" of his chest pain after sawing logs on a regular basis.

In the early part of this century, it was common practice to keep coronary patients in bed for prolonged periods of time and to curtail their level of physical activity markedly. Several Boston heart specialists were largely responsible for changing these old customs and traditions. In the 1950s, Sam Levine and Bernard Lown began to get patients with recent coronary attacks out of bed and into a chair and experienced no complications in so doing. Dr. Paul Dudley White gained national attention when he encouraged former President Eisenhower, himself a coronary patient, to be physically active as part of his coronary rehabilitation program. Over the past decade it has become an increasingly common practice to employ chair rest, early ambulation, and physical therapy in the medical management of the hospitalized coronary patient. The uncomplicated (i.e., no rhythm disturbances or heart failure) postcoronary patient is often released from the hospital after two to three weeks, and prior to discharge, has walked in the halls and up a flight of stairs under close medical supervision. Upon discharge, the patient may be given a schedule to follow at home for walking activities and flexibility exercises. At the end of several months, he or she will be eligible to participate in a medically supervised exercise program, of which there are now over eighty in the United States alone.

Medically supervised cardiac reconditioning centers were developed in the Bavarian region of Germany in 1954. During the late 1800s King Ludwig II converted Bavaria into a dreamland of breathtaking castles, strategically placed in the midst of the majestic Alps. In 1886 Ludwig drowned in the Starnberger Lake. Two years before Ludwig's tragic death a man named Max Beckmann was born in Leipzig and was later to become one of Germany's most famous painters. His son, Peter Beckmann, chose medicine as a career and established the first cardiac reconditioning center in the world in Ohlstadt, a small Bavarian community south of Munich. This center catered to the coronary-prone, rather than postcoronary patients. In 1959 Dr. Beckmann and several colleagues obtained permission to use the Castle Hohenried for a rehabilitation center. This castle, located on the opposite side of the lake where Ludwig II drowned, was the former home of a wealthy American, Wilhemina Busch Woods. Dr. Beckmann and his associate, Dr. Helmut Milz, accepted forty new patients at monthly intervals at the castle, and taught them how to take care of their hearts through proper exercise, diet, and self-relaxation. Gradually postcoronary patients were accepted at Hohenried when a modern 600-bed facility was opened in the mid-1960s, and at present at least two-thirds of the patients come for postcoronary disease rehabilitation.

Postcoronary rehabilitation

Rehabilitation of the postcoronary patient at Georgia Baptist Hospital begins on the day of admission to the intensive-care unit. Physical therapists begin a passive range of motion exercises in clinically stable patients and instructional programs on education concerning heart disease.

Two months after an attack patients return to the hospital gymnasium for intensive cardiac rehabilitation, consisting of dietary instruction, additional coronary risk factor education, and exercise therapy. The large gymnasium facility provides ample areas for jogging, volleyball, swimming, bowling, and a host of other activities (see Figure 17–1).

Figure 17–1 Postcoronary patients exercising in the hospital gymnasium.

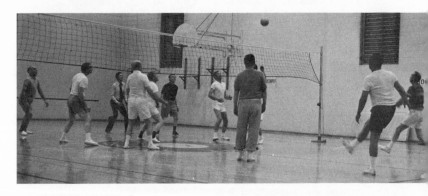

The program now consists of over 250 coronary patients who range in age from thirty to seventy. All patients must be referred to the program by their personal physician. The exercise sessions are each forty-five minutes long and are held three afternoons per week. Each session is broken down into fifteen-minute segments of walk-jog activity, flexibility exercises, and team sports. All sessions are supervised by a physician, nurse, and a physician's assistant, and the medical personnel generally exercise with the patients. A closed circuit television monitoring system keeps the various exercise areas under surveillance. Emergency resuscitation equipment, including an electrical defibrillator (see Figure 17–2) is immediately available and has been used on two occasions.

Figure 17–2 Defibrillator and emergency drug kit.

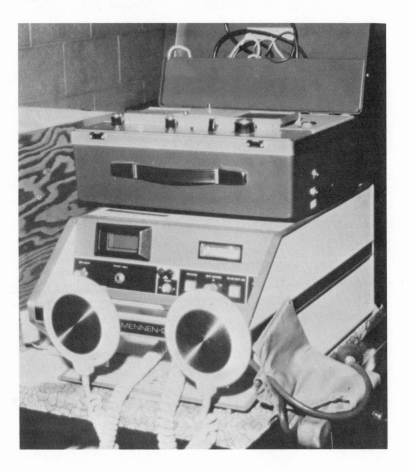

Each exercise session begins after the nurse records the blood pressure of every participant and inquires about the patient's present health. Patients exercise according to prescription cards and the latter are updated at two-to-three-week intervals. The physician in charge frequently exercises with the patients (see Figure 17–3).

Figure 17–3   The author (left) jogs with cardiac rehabilitation class members.

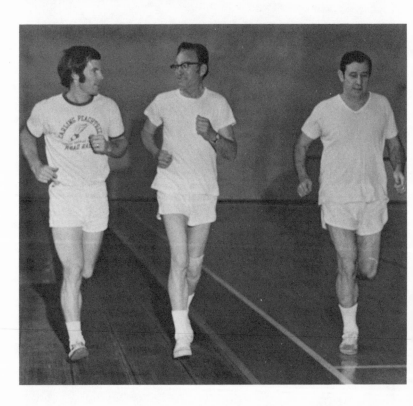

The highlight of the session is the volleyball game. The latter requires no special skills to be enjoyed. Competition is kept at a low level by altering the team members so that one is rarely on the same squad in a given month.

The Georgia Baptist program has been in operation for four years. During this time period there have been three deaths out of 250 patients from coronary disease (not temporally related to an exercise session), well below the expected rate of six to eight deaths per 100 patients each year. One death occurred in a man who had achieved a high degree of rehabilitation, only to give up his one-mile jog, to resume poor eating habits and cigarette consumption because of business pressures. Just prior to his death, he again expressed the desire to get back in shape, but unfortunately did not have the opportunity to do so.

The average participant in our gymnasium program will significantly improve his treadmill endurance time and his ability to utilize oxygen. His blood triglyceride level will decrease by 50 mg percent but the blood cholesterol level will not change appreciably in the absence of weight loss. His sense of well-being will be greatly enhanced, and almost all are able to return to gainful employment.

At present it is unclear whether such programs will prolong life and decrease the recurrence rates of coronary attacks. A National Exercise and Heart Disease Study, headed by a team of investigators from George Washington University, will attempt to answer these questions after data from the five-year study are tabulated. Until the latter are available it seems prudent to continue present trends in cardiac rehabilitation in view of the existing evidence which points to a variety of beneficial effects from such practices.

18

Prevention should start in childhood

On first glance, Muscatine, Iowa, and Scottsdale, Arizona, would not seem to have much in common. However, a closer look reveals that both communities are actively involved in aggressive coronary risk-factor screening in the pediatric age group. Under the sponsorship of the National Heart and Lung Institute, specialized centers of research in atherosclerosis (SCOR) have been established in various parts of the United States. Muscatine, located along the Mississippi River, has a population of 23,000 and was selected as a study site because of the stability of this population. Only 3 percent of the students in the school system drop out of the system in any given year. Over the past two years, 70 percent of the children in the public school system (4681 children, six to eighteen) have been screened for the risk factors of hypertension, hyperlipidemia, and obesity. Nearly 7 percent of the children had serum cholesterol levels in excess of 220 mg percent, well above the mean value for the group—182 mg percent. Serum triglyceride levels were elevated above 140 mg percent in 15 percent of the students, although this datum is less useful since the children ate breakfast prior to the test (ideally serum triglyceride levels should be obtained after a twelve-hour fast). High blood pressure levels were relatively uncommon in the group; no student under nine had levels in excess of 140/90 mm Hg, while 2.7 percent of the children above this age had elevated pressure readings. The frequency of obesity in the students was 12 percent, causing the administrators to reflect upon the nutritional and exercise habits in the school system. The potential scope of the project can be seen in the following example: The family of one youth with a Type II hyperlipidemia pattern (see Chapter 12) was evaluated in detail. Six of his seven siblings were found to have serum cholesterol levels between 270–300 mg percent. By checking out the families of each child who is found to have an abnormality, the total yield of the screening project could be enhanced tremendously.

The state of Arizona has undertaken a mammoth risk-factor screening program involving over 10,000 families of preschool children. Glenn Friedman of Scottsdale, a pediatrician, has been active in the project. Three years ago he established a cardiovascular intervention study within the framework of his private practice. The study involved checking the cholesterol and blood pressure levels of the children and their parents. The exercise tolerance of the former is checked on a stationary bicycle ergometer. The parents are queried as to their smoking habits. Guidelines are given as to methods of reducing the identified coronary risk factors. The families are encouraged to modify their intake of calories and of saturated fat. They are also advised to cut back on time spent in sedentary pursuits such as television viewing and to substitute family-type exercises such as hiking, swimming, and cycling.

There is an old adage that an ounce of prevention is worth a pound of cure. Assuming this to be true, would it not be worthwhile for us to intensify our efforts in the prevention of poor cardiovascular health habits in childhood rather than to spend all of our efforts in an attempt to change poor health habits in adults who already have severe coronary disease? Along these lines, what are the ways in which we can practice preventive cardiology in youngsters? It would seem prudent to begin by identifying children who have a high-risk factor for the development of premature coronary disease. The child whose parent or parents suffer from hypertension, diabetes, excessive blood lipids, or early heart attack falls in this category. So do children who manifest such findings as obesity, diabetes, hypertension, and hyperlipidemia.

In addition to the identification of high-risk children, efforts could be made in educating all school children about the nature of cardiovascular disease, the factors that seem responsible in part for the epidemic, and the ways in which such factors can be modified. Courses in preventive cardiology could be presented in health, science, or biology classes. Children could be taught to record blood pressures, as has been done in several Georgia school districts. They can be educated as to the perils of cigarette smoking, particularly when they reach the junior high school level when the urge to act big and to conform is so great.

The school nurse could routinely check blood pressures of all children and could administer brief questionnaires to both child and parents, seeking out the high-risk youngster. Physical education curricula need to be revised so that less emphasis is placed on team sports and more emphasis placed on learning individual endurance exercise skills (as tennis and swimming) that can provide enjoyment and enhanced physical fitness throughout a lifetime. Dietary programs for school lunches need to be revised so that a child at least has the opportunity to drink skim milk and eat margarine and extra lean beef if such is his or her upbringing.

While a great many things can be accomplished in schools, the majority of a child's habits are picked up at home. It is imperative that we review our own situations. Are we serving the right types of foods to our children, rather than encouraging them to snack on cookies and donuts? A son who rarely, if ever, sees his father in the pursuit of athletic endeavors will be an unlikely candidate for lifelong fitness habits himself. One only has to observe a group of children imitating their parents' cigarette smoking gestures to realize how such habits can literally be passed on from generation to generation.

What guidelines can a parent follow in order to begin preventive cardiology measures in childhood? Here a few recommendations:

1. Determine your own coronary risk factors by working closely with your physician. Begin at once to correct environmental practices, such as sedentary habits and sloppy dietary regimens, that will be of benefit to you and your children.

2. Ask your pediatrician to include a blood cholesterol and triglyceride check in your child's annual physical examination and inquire as to where cardiopulmonary fitness testing is carried out. In addition to following the weight of your child, the pediatrician might also follow the percentage of weight as fat, for a child of normal weight can have excessive body fat and insufficient lean body mass.

3. Seek membership in neighborhood clubs and organizations (such as the YMCA) that encourage family participation in physical fitness outings.

4. Encourage other parents and faculty members to make preventive health lectures part of the school curriculum. Enlist the support of your family physician in this endeavor.

We pass a lot of things on to the next generation, knowingly and unknowingly, some good and some bad. What a marvelous gift it would be, indeed, to pass on the example of lifelong health habits. Even if we acquire such habits late in life, perhaps too late to reap significant benefits for ourselves, it may still influence our children and our children's children to enjoy a longer and healthier life as a result of our efforts.

19

Preventive cardiology in practice

Up to this point, most of the sections in this book have been fragmented into a discussion of the various coronary risk factors. Let us now weave the individual strands together as we discuss the method and results of risk-factor detection, modification, and health enhancement in a private clinic.

Health assessment

At the Preventive Cardiology Clinic in Atlanta, Georgia, educational programs begin while the patient is in the waiting room. The books and magazines on the tables are lay publications pertaining to preventive cardiology and health maintenance. Slide-tape programs and video cassettes are also available on the various coronary risk factors.

A detailed medical history is obtained by the nurse and the physician, using the problem-oriented approach. Emphasis is placed on a meticulous family health history, looking for multiple family members who might have experienced signs of premature coronary heart disease. Exercise and dietary habits are carefully reviewed; the latter is accomplished by means of a three-day dietary history which the patient fills out and mails in to the nutritionist. While taking the history, the physician closely observes the patient, looking for signs of a Type A personality (Chapter 13) or other clues of excess stress and strain.

The physical examination is standard and includes prudent noncardiac screening techniques as tonometry (an eye test for glaucoma) and sigmoidoscopy (a rectal test) for those over forty. Body composition is measured by the skin-fold caliper technique, and body strength is estimated by using grip-strength devices.

Routine laboratory measurements, aside from the standard blood count and urinalysis, include assessment of serum cholesterol and triglyceride levels, blood sugar, chest X-ray, and the resting electrocardiogram. If the latter is unremarkable, the patient undergoes exercise stress testing on either the bicycle ergometer or the treadmill. Expired air is collected in plastic bags during the terminal phase of the exercise test in order to calculate the maximum amount of oxygen utilization. In addition to the latter, lung function is measured to look for early signs of emphysema. Another screening device is to measure the level of an enzyme known as alpha-1 antitrypsin in the blood. Low levels of this enzyme seem to enhance one's risk for developing emphysema. The last part of the evaluation involves psychological testing, ranging from the Minnesota Multiphasic Personality Inventory (MMPI) to screening tests for the Type A personality.

The level of physical fitness is plotted on a graph (see Figure 19–1), based on the oxygen utili-

Figure 19–1

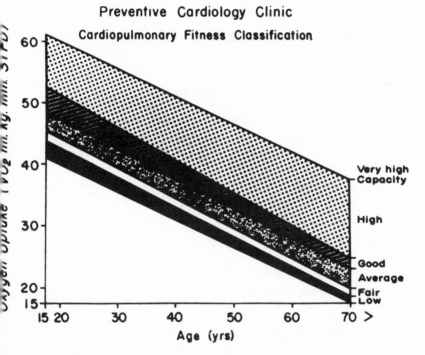

zation; the more fit a person is, the higher is his level of oxygen intake by the body. The risk of coronary disease is calculated by using the Coronary Risk Handbook, a publication of the American Heart Association. A problem list for each adverse health factor (see Figure 19–2) is compiled, and specific

Figure 19–2

Mr. D. West

COMPLETE PROBLEM LIST

DATE	ACTIVE	INACTIVE
3/6/74	(1) Low Cardiopulmonary Fitness →	
3/6/74	(2) Excess BODY FAT →	
3/6/74	(3) SUPRA-OPTIMAL BLOOD LIPIDS — a) Cholesterol - 285 mg/dl → b) Triglyceride - 175 mg/dl →	
3/6/74	(4) TYPE A PERSONALITY PATTERN	
3/6/74	(5) SYSTEMIC ARTERIAL HYPERTENSION →	
3/6/74	(6) FH of premature CHD	
3/6/74	(7) CIGARETTE SMOKING →	

recommendations are detailed for each problem. For instance, a specific diet is given for problems such as obesity or high blood cholesterol levels. Likewise, an exercise prescription is provided if the physical fitness chart does not reveal a high reading. The entire data base, including educational materials, is put together in booklet form (see Figure 19–3) and given to the patient. An important component of the data

Figure 19–3   A postcoronary patient's data-base booklet.

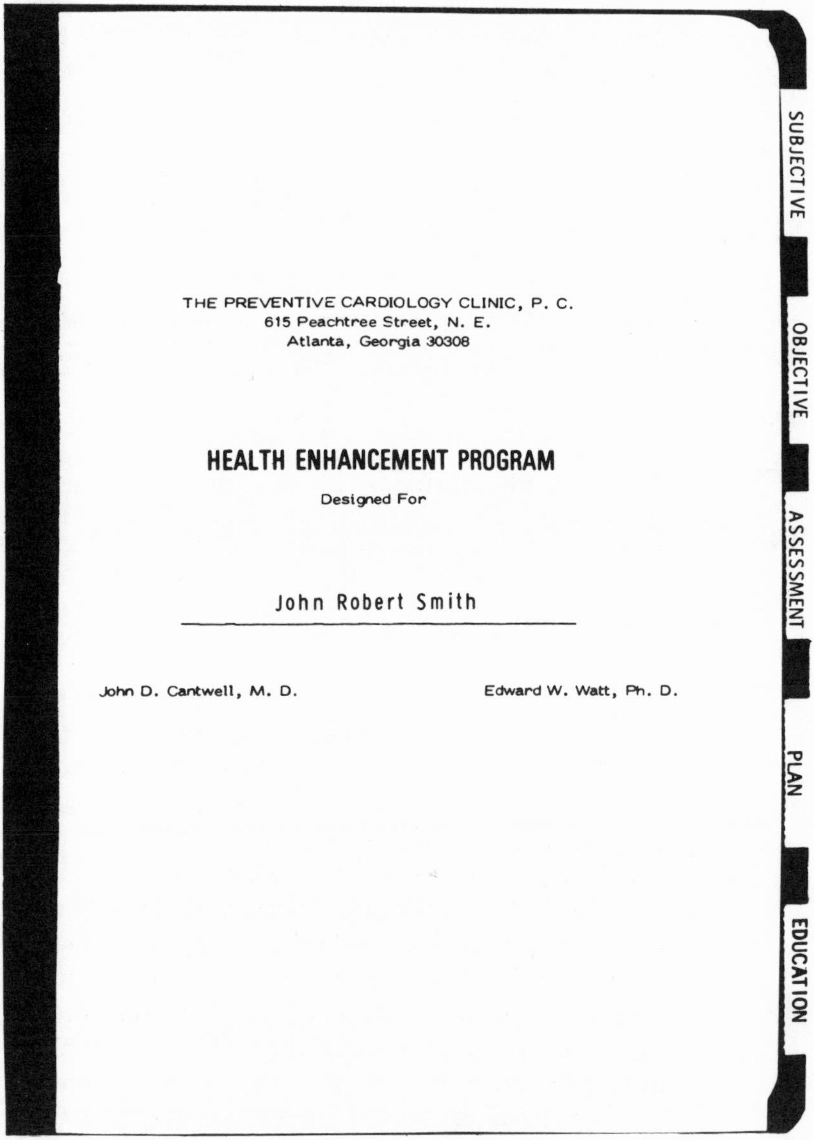

SUBJECTIVE

OBJECTIVE

ASSESSMENT

PLAN

EDUCATION

THE PREVENTIVE CARDIOLOGY CLINIC, P. C.
615 Peachtree Street, N. E.
Atlanta, Georgia 30308

HEALTH ENHANCEMENT PROGRAM

Designed For

John Robert Smith

John D. Cantwell, M. D.   Edward W. Watt, Ph. D.

booklet is the flow sheet (see Figure 19–4), which emphasizes the need for follow-up assessments and gives a patient the feeling that he is involved in his own health care.

Figure 19–4

HEALTH ENHANCEMENT PROGRESS FLOW SHEET

Date	Treadmill Test Time (minutes)	O₂ Uptake (ml/kg/min)	Weight	% Body Fat	Cholesterol	Triglyceride	Blood Pressure
1/29/73	6¾	35.0	224	19%	321	369	130/102
4/26/73	10	43.2	201	16%	283	153	140/90
8/3/73	11	48.5	192.5	12.7%	313	145	140/90
11/26/73	9¾	43.3	198	14%	294	106	140/90

Results

To date, data have been compiled on the first fifty-two patients who completed at least a six-month program in the cardiology clinic. Statistically significant improvements were seen in body composition—decreases in body fat (Figure 19–5), blood triglyceride levels (Figure 19–6), and blood pressure, and increases in the degree of physical fitness (Figure 19–7). Blood cholesterol levels did not show significant decreases although the average levels were not extremely elevated to begin with. While drug therapy could, no doubt, have appreciably lowered a number of these, I hesitate to use it in the

Figure 19–5   Decrease in body fat.

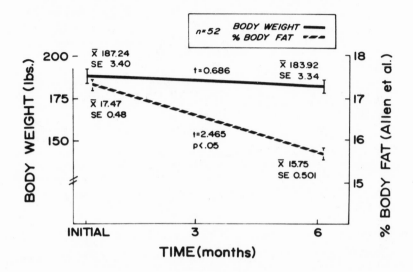

absence of very high cholesterol levels (over 300 mg percent) because of drug cost and occasional side effects.

While data on the cigarette smokers have not been officially tabulated, the initial impression is that at least 60–70 percent of the smokers either quit or markedly reduced their cigarette consumption after education and persuasion. It is difficult to measure changes in stress levels and modifications of personality. We have relied upon group dynamics for stress counseling, feeling that it is the hub of any approach to weight control, behavior modification, and antismoking regimens. From a purely subjective standpoint, almost all of the group have expressed an alleviation of considerable tension and anxiety,

**Figure 19–6 Decrease in blood triglyceride and
cholesterol levels.**

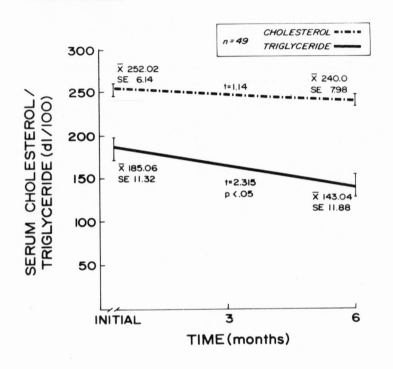

particularly after undergoing physical training. We
must await definitive test results, however, before
saying more.

Summary

There is nothing magical about the practice of preventive cardiology. It merely consists of
converting the vast amount of scientific data pertaining to this aspect of medicine into everyday usage. Why aren't physicians doing this? The answer

Figure 19–7 Increase in physical fitness.

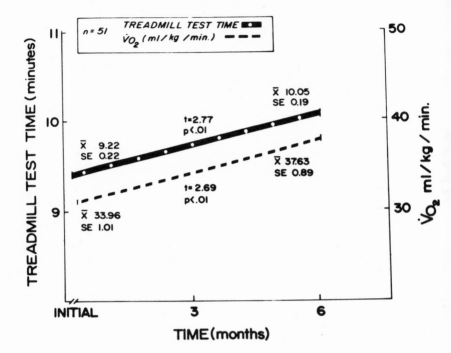

is that in many parts of the world they are, particularly in Europe and Scandinavia. In the United States it seems that we often get so bogged down taking care of sick people that we tend to neglect the well people. Another reason for the American lag in preventive cardiology is that our medical school curriculum is usually lacking in this topic.

Methods of preventive cardiology and health enhancement have been outlined in this chapter. For the most part, the ingredients can easily be incorporated by the practicing physician. While the results of such an approach seem very promising, additional large-scale studies are desirable. The lack of studies should not pose a stumbling block to the physician or to his patients, for common sense dictates the wisdom of many preventive health measures, such as moderation of living habits, apart from their effect on the cardiovascular system.

A letter from Paul Dudley White: His views on jogging and other exercises

I first met Doctor White at the Plaza Hotel in New York. The year was 1966. I was a medical intern, attending my first medical meeting in which he was the featured speaker. I was immediately impressed with his vitality as he charged up the stairs with his luggage, leaving me more than a little embarrassed in front of a crowded elevator.

Two years later, during a leisure moment in the vast Mayo Clinic Library, I happened upon a special issue of the American College of Cardiology in which former fellows of Doctor White shared their experiences and remembrances of the founding father of modern cardiology. It was fascinating reading and a fitting tribute to a man whose excellence in teaching and quest for knowledge was exceeded only by his dedication to primary patient care.

Figure 20–1   Letter from Dr. White.

PAUL DUDLEY WHITE, M. D.
264 BEACON STREET
BOSTON, MASS. 02116
CONSULTATION BY APPOINTMENT

December 18, 1968.

It is good to hear from you and to tell you of some of my thoughts and experiences with jogging. I have nothing against jogging as such if it is properly done, preferably outdoors in the open air and in pleasant surroundings, begun in youth and maintained throughout life. And its older participants should be carefully checked with a physician at hand when dealing with large numbers not adequately supervised, especially in dealing with respect to coronary patients or coronary candidates among the middle aged and elderly men who have not maintained a state of physical fitness throughout life.

I have personally known of two sudden deaths of middle-aged joggers while jogging around an indoor track and of a near death in a man who became a patient of mine with an acute coronary heart attack, and I presume that there have been others of whom I have not heard and who quite naturally would not be publicized. Hence I would prefer walking in the fresh air or safe cycling indoors or out for the middle aged or older – or swimming or other exercises that use the legs.

Running, squash, skiing, handball, and fast tennis are good for the young and can be maintained throughout life, with sensible and careful application to older adults if they are really fit and not candidates for coronary deaths.

Thus you can see that I have mixed feelings about jogging.

With best wishes, Paul D. White

The author thanks Mr. Roger Martin for permission to publish the letter from Doctor White.

As a cardiology fellow in San Diego, California, I became concerned about some of the sudden deaths and other cardiac complications which seemed to accompany the jogging craze. I discussed this with Mr. Roger Martin, the director of the Downtown YMCA in San Diego, and the latter sent an inquiry to the oracle himself—Paul Dudley White—to get his views. Doctor White's response, typically handwritten, is shown in Figure 20-1.

Doctor White was in favor of jogging for the younger age group, as long as it was "properly done" (presumably with prior medical clearance, adequate warm-up and cool down periods, and not accompanied by undue strain). He also advised other endurance exercise, such as squash, skiing, handball, and "fast tennis" for the young, pointing out that such activities can be maintained throughout life.

For the poorly conditioned middle-aged person, as well as the coronary-prone and postcoronary patient, Doctor White advised having a "physician at hand" for jogging activity. He favored walking "in the fresh air," indoor cycling, and swimming for these individuals, implying that these were safer forms of exercise than jogging.

Doctor White was a living testimony to the merits of lifelong vigorous activity. His encouragement of former President Eisenhower to resume his active life post-heart attack helped to change prevailing customs of prolonged bed rest for cardiac victims. His advice on jogging and other forms of exercise was sound and prevails, at least in our approach, to the use of exercise in the primary and secondary prevention of coronary heart disease.

21

Summary

Coronary heart disease of near epidemic magnitude has become the major health problem in the United States and in various other countries of the world. Unless we modify our current lifestyle, 40 percent of the readers of this book will succumb to this disease.

While major advances have been made and will continue to be made in the diagnosis and treatment of coronary disease, the final answer will undoubtedly lie in prevention. For prevention to be effective, it must begin in childhood since there is ample evidence that the disease process starts early. Coronary risk factors have been identified. Undoubtedly additional factors will be identified in the years to come. However, while we are awaiting the final answer, it is imperative that we apply the information already at hand in countering this epidemic. Application likewise must begin in childhood but can be adapted at almost any age. Our children should be screened for blood fat abnormalities (such as hypercholesterolemia) and hypertension. Their level of physical fitness should be ascertained, either by the Cooper 12-minute field test or by exercise stress testing. Children must be taught how to eat properly, establishing eating habits that will carry through to later life. They must also be taught various forms of physical skills that they can enjoy throughout life, not just participating in team sports in school.

Sedentary living is a coronary risk factor. Unlike blood pressure and cholesterol measurements, it is often difficult to quantify. Largely for this reason, studies are often conflicting as to its relative importance. Studies in animals and in humans, however, show a strong trend toward the beneficial effects of exercise training on the cardiovascular system. Since exercise is inexpensive and safe, we need to make greater use of it in our attack against premature coronary heart disease. While exercise training will continue to be useful in treating coronary patients, we need to start thinking before the fact, rather than afterward, and to apply exercise in that context, along with other measures of preventive cardiology. We have a lot to gain by this approach.

Glossary

Angina pectoris — chest discomfort, usually brought on by activity or emotional upset, reflecting inadequate blood supply of heart muscle.

Arteriography — the technique in which dye is injected through a thin tube (catheter) into arteries so that the latter can be visualized by X-ray methods.

Atherosclerosis — a disease process in which fatty material such as cholesterol deposits in the lining of arteries.

Bicycle ergometer — a stationary bicycle with varying speed and resistance used in laboratories for exercise testing.

Blood platelets — a circular disc-like component found in the blood of all mammals and concerned with blood clotting.

Bruce treadmill method — a standard protocol of exercise testing on a treadmill device wherein the speed and slope of the treadmill are elevated at three-minute intervals.

Carboxyhemoglobin — carbon monoxide which is attached to red blood cells.

Catecholamines — a group of compounds similar to adrenalin found in the adrenal gland and in nerve endings.

Catheterization — the technique of inserting a catheter into an artery or vein for purposes of measuring pressure and of injecting dye into the heart or large arteries.

Cholesterol — a fatty substance found in all animal fats and oils and in foods such as egg yolks, whole milk, butter, and cheese.

Chylomicron — fatty particles which are found in the blood after digestion of fat.

Coronary plaques — deposits of fatty substances in the lining of arteries.

Coronary vasodilator — a drug which results in widening or dilatation of coronary arteries.

Defibrillator — a machine which can deliver a strong electrical charge to the heart.

Diastolic blood pressure — the pressure of blood within the arteries during the relaxation phase of the heart cycle (which alternates contraction and relaxation).

Ectomorph — an individual with a tall, thin body build.

Electrocardiogram — the technique of recording the electrical activity of the heart.

Endomorph — an individual with an excess of fatty tissue.

Epidemiology — the study of the nature of a disease process, particularly factors related to cause.

Epinephrine — a substance produced in the adrenal gland which increases blood pressure and accelerates heart rate.

Hyperlipidemia — elevated levels of fat in the circulating blood.

Hypertension — increased pressure of blood within the arteries exceeding 140 mm Hg during heart contraction (systole) and 90 mm Hg during heart relaxation (diastole).

Hypothalamus — a region of the brain having to do with control of such entities as appetite, body temperature, and sleep.

Ischemia — a state of inadequate blood supply to body tissue.

Lipoprotein — a combination of fat and protein which circulates in the blood stream.

Mesomorph — an individual with a short, muscular build.

MET unit — a measure of the body's caloric (or energy) expenditure; one MET unit is the amount of energy burned in the resting state (expresed in calories used per minute).

Mitochondria — the structure in a body cell concerned with energy production.

Monoglyceride — a single fatty acid which is connected to glycerol, an oil made in the body.

Myocardial infarction — destruction of heart muscle cells because of inadequate blood supply.

Saphenous vein grafts — the surgical technique where a leg vein (saphenous vein) is removed and sewn into the heart forming a "detour" for coronary blood flow around a blocked artery.

Saturated fat — animal fat that is in solid form at room temperature.

Sigmoidoscopy — inspection of the lower bowel through a long speculum inserted into the rectum.

Skinfold caliper technique — a measure of body fat using a tension caliper device; skinfold thickness is measured in various body sites.

Small bowel bypass — a surgical technique which decreases food absorption by rerouting food passage in the bowel.

Somatotypes — categories of body builds.

Sphygmomanometer — a cuff device which is applied to the arm to measure blood pressure.

Systolic — pertaining to events taking place during the contraction of the heart.

Thrombosis — the formation of a clot in a blood vessel.

Thrombus — a plug or clot in a blood vessel.

Tonometry — the technique of measuring the pressure within the eye.

Triglyceride — three fatty acids which are bound to glycerol, an oil made in the body.

Unsaturated fat — fat, usually in the form of vegetable oil, that is in liquid form at room temperature.

Ventricular fibrillation — chaotic electrical activity of the heart.

Ventromedial nucleus — an area of the hypothalamus in the brain which signals the body when enough food has been eaten.

Index

as a risk factor in heart
disease, 7, 8, 11
in test patients, 14–15
tests on, 14–15
Hiller, John, 88
Hirsch, Dr. Jules, on fat
cell theory of
obesity, 142
Hohenreid Castle
(Bavaria), 155
Horseback riding, 58, 59
Horseshoe pitching, 58
Houdini, Harry, 91
Hunza (Kashmere),
longevity of persons
in, 91
Hypercholesterolemia, 182
Hyperlipidemia, in
children, 162
Hypertension
causes of, 103–4
in children, 162, 182
as a coronary risk
factor, 15, 101–9
Hypertrophy, cardiac
enlargement due to, 80
Hypothalamus region
of the brain, 140–41

Ibrahim, Dr. M. A., on
hostility level as a risk
factor in heart
disease, 124
Ice skating, 58, 62

Inderal, for treatment of
heart muscle, 4
Irish, coronary disease
among the, 9
Ironshell, Indian chief, 89–90
Ischemia, defined, 34
Isometric exercise, 55
Isordil, for treatment of
chest pain, 4
Italian American
community at Roseto,
Pa., heart disease
studies in, 122–23
Italy, studies of heart
disease in, 10

Japan, studies of heart
disease in, 10–11
Jogging, 59, 65

Kelley, Johnny, 88
Keys, Dr. Ancel
on behavior patterns and
heart disease, 124
study on heart disease
and death rate by, 10
Kidneys, and
hypertension, 107
Koch, Edward, and walk-jog
regimen, 65
Kopcha, Dr. Joe, 89
Kritchevsky, David, poem
on sexual activity and
heart condition, 134